Medical
Note
Mastery

Primary Care and
Emergency Department
Scribe Edition

Tayler Diedrichsen
Laura Bultman, MD
MEDICAL NOTE MASTERS, LLC | MINNEAPOLIS, MN

Medical Note Mastery

Primary Care and Emergency Department Scribe Edition

©2021, Medical Note Masters, LLC

ISBN 9798675122059

www.medicalscribetraining.net
admin@mednotemasters.com

Printed in the USA

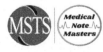

We would like to dedicate this volume to the many scribes and physicians we have had the pleasure of working with over the years. It has been an honor to be a part of helping you in your medical career.

The art of medicine consists of amusing the patient while nature cures the disease. -Voltaire

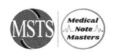

Table of Contents

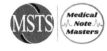

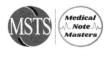

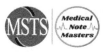

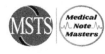

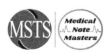

1. Introduction

The Medical Scribe Role

Up until the 1990s, medical scribes did not exist to much extent. Healthcare providers documented notes by hand, which were often illegible. With the "tech boom" in the 1990s and the advance of computing and the internet, it became appealing to use technology to record and share patient information. With more data being recorded, more regulatory agencies began to collect data and associate data with reimbursement. To incentivize the use of electronic health records (EHRs), government payors began offering subsidies to organizations that adopted them. However, there was a catch to obtaining these funds: medical documentation needed to include even more components. Healthcare providers became more and more frustrated with how much time they spent on charts, so the scribe industry began.

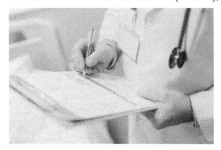

The medical scribe's primary role is to record the detailed information from a patient's clinic visit into the electronic chart. First and foremost, this allows the healthcare provider to focus on patients and save hours of charting after each shift. Using scribes can significantly reduce the time delay for documentation to get into the EHR, helping patient care. In some settings, clinics utilize medical assistants or other roles to contribute to documentation, so sometimes scribes are simply called "documentation assistants" since various healthcare roles may participate in note documentation.

Despite their widespread use, scribes do not yet have a licensed role defined by a national regulatory body, as a medical assistant or nurse does. The Joint Commission, a predominant authority that accredits hospitals, neither supports nor discourages scribes, but recommends that scribes are adequately trained and that organizations who use scribes have well-defined local policies. In some cases, other healthcare roles may also function as documentation assistants, so the restrictions listed below may not apply. Local clinic policies vary, so what may be allowed or disallowed in a particular setting cannot be precisely predicted. However, there are some generalities to follow.

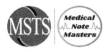

Medical scribes are responsible for performing the following actions:

✓ Documenting patient interviews and examinations in the health record while they are performed by the provider or immediately afterward

✓ Assisting the provider with the review of previous notes or labs or finding other useful information in the EHR

✓ Updating medical, social and other histories

✓ Documenting all performed elements of the physical exam

✓ Documenting procedures and treatments performed by the provider

✓ Documenting the patient's clinical progress during the visit

✓ Transcribing ancillary test results, including laboratory, imaging, and EKG results and the provider's interpretation of these results

✓ Documenting the physician's consultations with other physicians and family members

✓ Accurately inputting diagnoses as directed by the provider

✓ Writing the final clinical decision making and assessment dictated by the provider

✓ Documenting the complete follow-up plan, including instructions for patients including follow-up indications clearly and without ambiguity

✓ Alerting the physician if a patient's chart is incomplete

✓ Assisting with medication reconciliation documentation

What else is expected of a medical scribe?

✓ Be prepared and on time to your shift

✓ Dress appropriately to the local clinical attire

✓ Respect patient privacy

✓ Respect the sensitivity of medical issues discussed

✓ Type quickly and accurately

✓ Make use of downtime

✓ Proactively seek out the physician's activities

✓ Take the time to learn and ask questions

1. Introduction

Scribes are PROHIBITED from performing the following actions:

- ⊘ Interviewing patients or family members
- ⊘ Examining patients
- ⊘ Independently making medical decisions or giving medical advice
- ⊘ Transcribing medical decisions without direct guidance
- ⊘ Assisting with medical procedures, specimen collection, IV placement, or any other lab or nursing duties
- ⊘ Any physical interaction with a patient beyond a handshake, such as rolling the patient on the exam table, changing linens, or assisting with ambulation
- ⊘ Logging into the EHR as a physician or anyone else
- ⊘ In most cases, entering orders into the EHR (depending on local policy)
- ⊘ Signing or approving orders
- ⊘ Relaying verbal orders to nursing staff
- ⊘ Signing medical notes, either manually or electronically
- ⊘ Phoning in orders, prescriptions, or refills
- ⊘ Serving as a medical translator

Most medical scribes are current or recent college students that are using the job as a steppingstone to medical, physician assistant, public health, or nursing school. Many scribes find that they gain an extensive, practical foundation of knowledge that will serve them throughout their medical career. Learning the materials in this manual and then applying them in the real world of medicine will provide you with a significant jumpstart in your medical education. When the rest of your medical or nursing school classmates are struggling to write a medical note, as a proficient scribe, you will be able to focus on learning the medicine.

The medical scribe's role is difficult to define precisely, as it can vary between providers and settings. In the end, your goal is to be able to document the history in an organized fashion, record the physical accurately using proper terminology, and transcribe the assessment and plan based on the provider's discussion with you and the patient. Over time a skilled scribe can learn the provider's preferences and thought process, gaining valuable medical rationale knowledge, and often a mentor-student relationship is forged. We hope that your journey to becoming a scribe will lead to invaluable clinical experience!

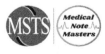

HIPAA and Patient Privacy

Scribes function in a sensitive medical environment and are exposed to private information regarding patients and families. While it is commonplace to discuss what happened at work with friends and family, never include any information that could identify the patient or the specific incident.

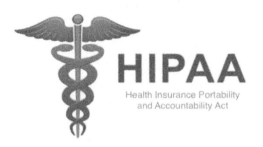

The single most significant confidentiality law in healthcare is known as HIPAA (pronounced hip-uh). This term often incites fear by its very mention due to its associated fines and penalties. HIPAA stands for the Health Insurance Portability and Accountability Act. In 1996, this federal legislation created national standards for how patient health information can be used and shared. HIPAA, the Health Information Technology for Economic and Clinical Health (HITECH) Act of 2009 and additional local laws create comprehensive privacy obligations for healthcare providers and staff. All healthcare workers must understand HIPAA legislation's essential components, and most facilities require a formal training session before allowing EHR access. Here we cover the privacy rules that scribes need to know.

HIPAA generally protects what is known as Protected Health Information (PHI), which encompasses a broad list of any data that the patient discloses to the clinic that could be used to identify that patient.

Table 1.1: Common examples of PHI

Name	Any other piece of information that would allow
Date of birth	indirect identification, such as "I can't say who the
Medical record number	patient was, but he's the manager at the gas station."
Address	
Email address	A car accident occurs, and the driver is named on the
Phone number	news. You cannot tweet, "The driver turned out to be
Images	diabetic! I am so sad for his family."

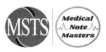

1. Introduction

Scribes are administrative members of the healthcare team with access to multiple PHI elements, so even though scribes do not provide healthcare, they must still adhere to basic HIPAA tenets outlined below.

- Only staff members involved in the treatment of a specific patient should access that patient's record. It may be tempting to open a patient's chart in the ER or clinic with an interesting chief complaint or a famous name, but opening the chart out of curiosity is a privacy violation. Other infringements in this category include looking at medical records for family members' medical records, friends, neighbors, coworkers, etc.

- The minimum number of people should access the minimum necessary amount of information for the required clinical task. If a gastroenterologist is consulted, that physician will access the chart but it would be unlikely that 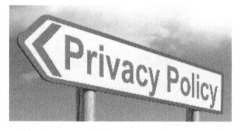 the entire clinic staff would need to read every clinical note. Similarly, for a patient with a gastrointestinal bleed, it is unnecessary to view previous marital therapy notes that are irrelevant. To technologically assist with compliance in this category, most EHRs are set up so that different login credentials have different information access levels. For example, front desk scheduling personnel might not be able to view full patient note details, only the reason for visit.

- Any unwarranted disclosure of protected health information is an infraction of HIPAA policy, called a "breach." Healthcare entities are required by the HIPAA and HITECH acts to create systems to physically and technologically prevent PHI breaches. Despite creating robust IT protections, however, humans can easily breach confidentiality even without malicious intent.
  - For example, the clinic schedule lists a scribe's cousin's name for a prenatal care visit. The scribe cannot post online "Congratulations Sue!" or text her husband, "I'm so excited for you guys!"
  - If a local athlete is seen in the ER, scribes cannot announce to friends what a relief it is that the quarterback didn't break his leg.
  - Social media is likely the single riskiest area, so think twice before posting ANYTHING work-related.

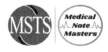

Okay to share PHI with colleagues involved in the care of the patient

Not okay to share PHI on social media, friends, or family

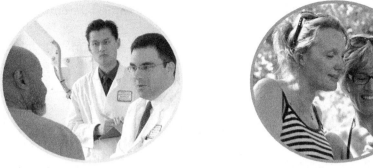

- It is best practice to avoid printing anything from the EHR, but any piece of paper containing PHI must be disposed of in a secure waste bin rather than a regular trash can. These bins are professionally shredded.

- Although a patient may have charts with multiple organizations, patients must consent to transfer information from one healthcare entity to another. Scribes may need to enter some of these "outside" records into the current chart.

- In emergency scenarios, PHI may be accessed without patient consent when necessary for treatment purposes or to prevent a threat to others. PHI may also rarely be used without permission if a person or the public is under an imminent health threat, and the disclosure might prevent harm. Examples include a psychiatrist learning of a patient's plan to harm someone and notifying the police, or a clinic disclosing a reportable infectious disease to the department of health.

- As outlined by HIPAA, these rules apply to all past, present, and future patient charts and are not limited to protected health information found within EHRs.

- Within most healthcare venues, other patients and bystanders may be in waiting areas or hallways, so it can be unwise to use a patient's full name in conversation. As a rule of thumb, while in earshot of others, reference a patient by a room number or condition rather than a full name to avoid any inadvertent breaches of confidentiality.

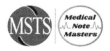

1. Introduction

For the patient's benefit, HIPAA also formally granted patients access to their own medical records. Patients may access limited sets of data via EHR portals, which are formatted to be more patient-friendly, or they may request the entirety of their chart. Documentation assistants are not often involved in the process, but they do need to be cognizant that what is entered into the medical record may be later viewed by the patient or other parties like attorneys. With this in mind, documentation language must remain professional.

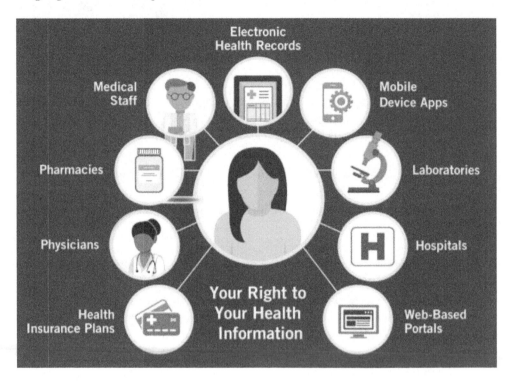

Generally, the IT department builds an infrastructure so that PHI is protected from outside hackers and internal leaks such as printing and screenshots. However, humans can make serious IT mistakes that compromise PHI.

Do NOT:

- ⊘ Share usernames or passwords
- ⊘ Write passwords on sticky notes or store them on any device without strong password-protection

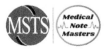

- ⊘ Leave PHI like the day's schedule in plain sight
- ⊘ Allow inappropriate persons to see the computer screen
- ⊘ Leave the computer unattended while signed-in to the EHR
- ⊘ Save printouts or screenshots
- ⊘ Connect to the EHR via an unsecured or public wireless network like a coffee shop
- ⊘ Save PHI on personal devices

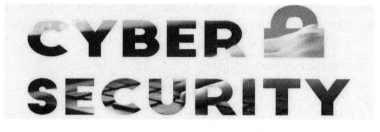

Last but not least, when in doubt, ask a supervisor! HIPAA requires that facilities have a privacy officer in charge of monitoring compliance, and that expert can address more specific concerns.

End of Chapter Quiz

1. Which of the following is considered PHI?
    a. Patient's name
    b. Patient's phone number
    c. Patient's address
    d. All of the above
2. Which of the following actions is a scribe prohibited from performing?
    a. Documenting all performed elements of the physical exam
    b. Writing the final clinical decision making and assessment dictated by the provider
    c. Relaying verbal orders to nursing staff
    d. Alerting the physician if a patient's chart is incomplete
3. PHI can never be accessed without a patient's consent.
    a. True
    b. False
4. What does PHI stand for?
    a. Protected health information
    b. Patient heart information
    c. Protected human information
    d. Patient health information
5. Scribes are certified just like other healthcare providers.
    a. True
    b. False
6. Since scribes are a nationally-standardized role, scribe positions are the same from one employer to another.
    a. True
    b. False
7. To be on the safe side, scribes should avoid discussing work-related topics on social media.
    a. True
    b. False

Answers: 1. D 2. C 3. B 4. A 5. B 6. B 7. A

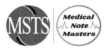

2. Medical Terminology

This chapter has two major parts: terminology related to anatomy and kinesiology, and terminology broken down into its root pieces. These two sections form the foundation of medical terminology and allow accurate and concise descriptions of the human body for physical exam documentation. Depending on the medical specialty, the amount of terminology required for documentation varies greatly, as one might expect if comparing psychiatry to sports medicine. We intend to set some groundwork, but most documentation assistants will acquire additional terminology on-the-job.

General Anatomy and Kinesiology

The study of the human body and movement, respectively, is called anatomy and kinesiology, and these terms are vital in medical practice. Many of the terms in this section exist in pairs, in which one word is used in relation to another word or in relation to an anatomic landmark.

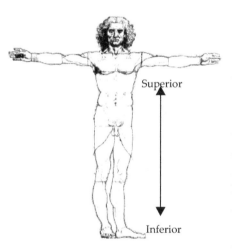

Figure 2.1: Superior vs. Inferior

Superior vs. Inferior
Superior means "above" and inferior means "below" in medical parlance. The most superior part of the body is the top of the head, and the most inferior part of the body is the foot (as shown in Figure 2.1). Like many other medical terms, this pair of terms is used to describe two landmarks relative to each other. For example, the chest is superior to the abdomen but inferior to the head. Depending on the subject of the sentence, either term may be appropriate.

For example:
• The eyebrows are *superior* to the eyes.
• The eyes are *inferior* to the eyebrows.

Proximal vs. Distal

When describing the location of something on an *extremity*, the terms proximal and distal are used instead of superior and inferior. The term "extremity" refers to an arm or leg. Proximal means closer to the origin (starting point) of an extremity. The shoulder is located at the proximal upper extremity, and the hip is located at the proximal lower extremity. In contrast, distal means farther from the origin of an extremity. The fingers are located at the distal upper extremity, and the toes are located at the distal lower extremity. Again, these terms are used when describing the extremities and do not apply to the trunk.

For example:

- The laceration is 2 cm distal to the olecranon (point of the elbow)

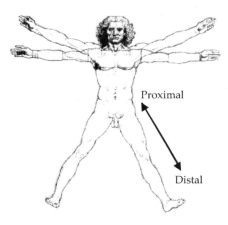

Figure 2.2: Proximal vs. Distal

Medial vs. Lateral

Another essential concept is medial versus lateral. Medial means closer to the midline of the body, and lateral means further from the midline. These terms can be absolute or relative. For example, the medial ankle is the inside part of the ankle (closer to the imaginary midline of the body). Or, a finding can be medial or lateral to an anatomical structure (such as a laceration lateral to the left eyebrow). Medial and lateral can generally be applied to any part of the body including the finger, foot, leg, head, chest—mostly everywhere. In Figure 2.3, medial and lateral are outlined on the patient's trunk and right lower extremity.

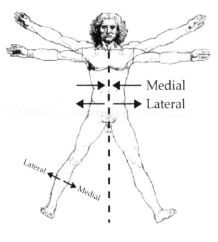

Figure 2.3: Medial vs. Lateral

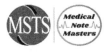

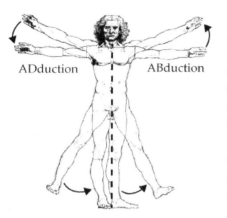

Figure 2.4: Abduction vs. Adduction

ABduction vs. ADduction

Abduction and adduction refer to the movement of an extremity around a ball and socket joint (i.e., shoulders and hips) and are shown in Figure 2.4. Adduction is movement of an extremity toward the midline of the body. Abduction is movement away from the midline. Because these terms sound very similar, you may hear them pronounced "A-dee-duction" and "A-bee-duction." An excellent way to remember this is that abduction means "to take away," as in the arms being taken further away from the midline of the body.

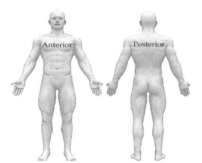

Figure 2.5: Anterior vs. Posterior

Anterior vs. Posterior

Anterior refers to the front of the body or the front side of a body part. Posterior refers to the back of the body or backside of a body part. Note that in proper anatomical diagrams, like Figure 2.5, the palms of the hands are facing forward and are thus considered anterior. Inversely, the back of the hand is therefore the posterior aspect.

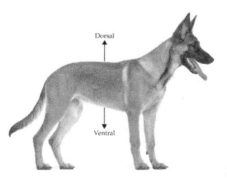

Figure 2.6: Dorsal vs. Ventral

Dorsal vs. Ventral (and Volar)

The hands and feet are often described by terms other than anterior and posterior. The nomenclature for these terms dates back to four-legged vertebrate anatomy. When describing these animals, we use the terms dorsal and ventral rather than posterior and anterior, respectively. Dorsal is similar to posterior and means towards the back. Ventral is similar to anterior and means towards the front.

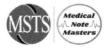

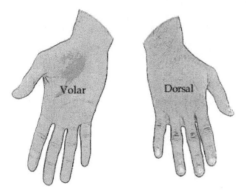

Figure 2.7: Volar vs. Dorsal

Due to standard anatomic positioning, as pictured in Figure 2.5, the top of the hands and feet is described as "dorsal" because they point dorsally in this standard position. Likewise, the palm of the hands and soles of the feet are defined as the ventral aspect. However, since patients are seldom in "standard" position, the palms of the hands are usually described as the volar aspect rather than the ventral aspect (Figure 2.7).

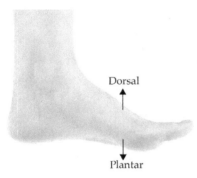

Figure 2.8: Dorsal vs. Plantar

The sides of the feet are labeled similarly to the hands with the terms dorsal and ventral. However, the ventral aspect, also known as the sole of the foot, is more commonly documented as the plantar aspect (Figure 2.8). For example:

- 2mm puncture wound on plantar aspect left foot, medial aspect approximately 1 cm distal to MTP joint.

Abdominal Regions

Since many of the previous terms only apply to the extremities (proximal, distal, etc.), we still need to outline the medical terms used to describe the trunk of the body, particularly the abdomen. The abdomen is the region on the anterior body surface overlying the abdominal organs. It has multiple landmarks and, first and foremost, is divided into four quadrants, including:

RUQ	right upper quadrant
LUQ	left upper quadrant
LLQ	left lower quadrant
RLQ	right lower quadrant

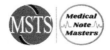

In the abdomen, the umbilicus ("belly button") is the dividing point for upper and lower quadrants and the left from the right. The flanks are the regions on the lateral abdomen that connect the abdomen to the back. Note that left and right always refer to the *patient's* left and right, from the patient's perspective.

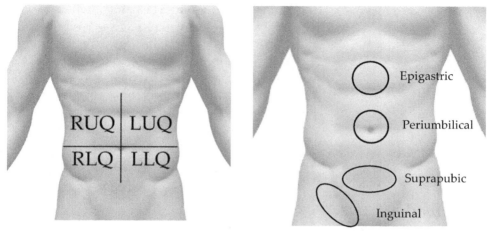

Figure 2.9: Abdominal quadrants   Figure 2.10: Abdominal regions

Patients may complain of abdominal pain which is neither right- nor left-sided. For these cases, the terms epigastric, periumbilical, and suprapubic help describe the appropriate region. Epigastric refers to the central upper abdomen, referring to "gastric" which means stomach. Periumbilical refers to the umbilicus area, often the area where children rub their tummy to indicate pain location. The suprapubic region is the area just above (or superior to) the pubic bone. The inguinal area is the low crease where the abdomen meets the upper leg, often called the "groin," and may be associated with musculoskeletal strains or an abdominal issue such as a hernia. If a patient is completely unable to localize the pain, then the term "generalized" may be used.

For example:
- Positive diffuse tenderness in upper abdomen, maximal in RUQ
- Well-healed, oblique linear scar in RLQ
- Positive abdominal wall defect palpable at umbilicus, approximately 2 cm in diameter. Positive bulge with cough with immediate reduction.
- Positive LAD in R inguinal fold, firm round mobile 1 cm mass with overlying erythema. Pulse 2+. No bulge with Valsalva.

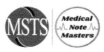

Basic Skeletal Anatomy

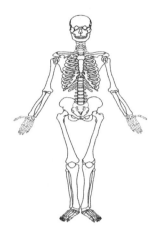

The typical adult has over 200 bones. Most of these are unnecessary to memorize at this point in your medical career, but there are several bones and articulations (i.e. joints) that you should be familiar with as a scribe. The following section will provide an overview of the major bones and joints that are essential to your knowledge. Many of these anatomical terms serve as valuable landmarks for describing the location of a patient's pain or injury (in combination with the terms just covered) and are frequently used in documentation. These terms serve as a foundation for scribe work as well as for medical training as a whole. We will begin from top to bottom, in the conventional fashion.

The Head

Four major cranial regions overlie the skull bones, which include:

- **Frontal** bone – this single bone makes up the forehead.

- **Parietal** bones – these two symmetric bones lie on either side of the skull midline of the skull i.e. the sagittal suture.

- **Temporal** bones – the temporal bones form the areas around each ear and are part of the skull base. This region protects the vestibulocochlear complex (balance and hearing centers), and several facial nerves.

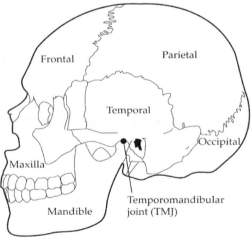

Figure 2.11: Cranial and facial bones

- **Occipital** bone – this single bone forms the posterior of the skull. It is a common region for head trauma after falling.

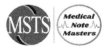

Additional facial bones to note are the:

- **Maxillary** bones (*singular maxilla, plural maxillae*) – these two bones comprise the upper jaw. The upper teeth are embedded in the maxilla.

- **Mandible** – the lower jaw or mandible is the large bone that hinges at the temporal bone. The lower teeth are embedded in the mandible.

- **Zygoma/Zygomatic arch** – the "cheekbone"

The main joint to know is the **temporomandibular joint (TMJ)** – the articulation of the mandible and temporal bone, connected by ligaments that stretch and allow the jaw to open and close. It is a common site for inflammatory pain and clicking.

The Thorax

The bones of the thorax protect vital body organs (heart, lungs, liver, kidneys, etc.). Minor trauma may cause a musculoskeletal injury, while significant trauma may result in damage to the internal organs. You will most frequently encounter this terminology during the physical exam, as the physician describes abnormal findings (e.g., "The patient is exquisitely tender over the right AC joint").

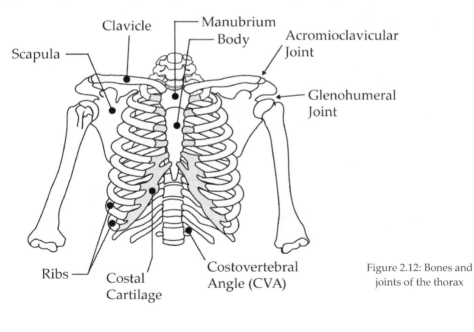

Figure 2.12: Bones and joints of the thorax

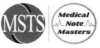

- Clavicles – these two bones connect medially to the sternum and laterally to the acromion of the scapula, forming the acromioclavicular (AC) joint.

- Humerus – the upper arm bone that articulates with the scapula to form the shoulder joint.

- Scapula – also known as the shoulder blade, the scapulae (plural) form the flat bones on each side of the upper back. It includes the underlying "socket" (the glenoid fossa) that makes up the ball-and-socket joint of the shoulder. It also connects to the clavicles via the acromion process, forming the acromioclavicular (AC) joint.

- Ribs – there are 12 thoracic ribs (corresponding to the 12 thoracic vertebrae), 10 of which connect to the sternum and form the protective cavity for the heart and lungs. The remaining inferior two ribs are called "floating ribs" because they do not connect directly to the sternum.

- Sternum – the sternum is made of three parts, including the manubrium (the top part), the body (the middle), and the xiphoid (the small point at the bottom). It connects to the clavicles superiorly (at the clavicular notches) and the ribs laterally via the costal cartilage.

- Costal cartilage – this is the region where the ribs connect to the sternum via cartilage. This area may become inflamed, painful, and tender—a condition called costochondritis ("chondral" refers to cartilage, "costal" to the ribs, and "itis" to inflammation).

- Costovertebral angle (CVA) – the region formed by the junction of the inferior ribs and corresponding vertebrae (T12) in the mid-back. This is an important region, as each kidney lies partly below the CVA, kidney problems may result in tenderness to percussion of this region.

- Acromioclavicular (AC) joint – the connection of the clavicle to the anterior process of the scapula, called the acromion process. This joint is commonly injured or "separated" from sports injuries and may develop a lump.

- Glenohumeral joint – the shoulder ball-and-socket joint formed by the head of the humerus and glenoid fossa of the scapula.

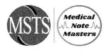

The Upper Extremities

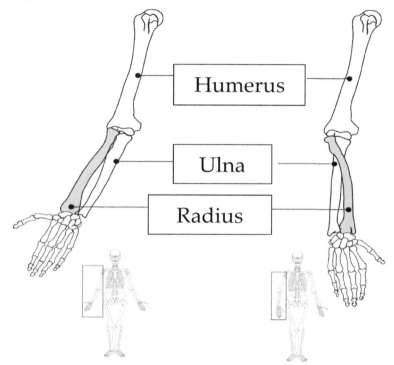

Figure 2.13: Radius and ulna of right arm in supinated (left) and pronated (right) positions

The bones of the upper extremities are similar to the lower extremities in that there is one large bone in the proximal aspect and two smaller bones in the distal aspect. The forearm bones (radius and ulna) are somewhat more troublesome because they rotate around each other with supination/pronation movements. In standard anatomical positioning, the palms are facing forward (left side of Figure 2.14), so the radius is on the lateral aspect, and the ulna is on the medial aspect of the forearm. However, with the palms facing posteriorly, technically known as a pronated position, the radius is on the medial aspect, and the ulna is on the lateral aspect (right side of Figure 2.14). For this reason, it is less common to describe something as "over the medial forearm" because it is too easy to mix up which way the hand was turned. Instead, the radius and ulna are used as landmarks when describing the location of something on the forearm, because they are more consistent. For a laceration, you may hear it described as "over the radial aspect of the distal forearm," indicating it is on the thumb-side of the forearm near the wrist.

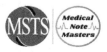

- **Humerus** – the upper arm bone that articulates with the scapula to form the shoulder joint. Distally, it forms the elbow joint, where it connects with the radius and ulna.

- **Radius** – the forearm bone that is straight when the forearm is supinated (left side of Figure 2.14) but rotates around the ulna with pronation of the forearm (right side of Figure 2.14). The radius connects to the wrist at the thumb side of the hand, and the radial pulse is palpated just proximal to the volar wrist crease on the thumb side of the forearm.

- **Ulna** – the forearm bone that forms the primary connection to the humerus and thus, the elbow joint.

- **Olecranon** – the protuberant proximal end of the ulna forming the pointy part of the elbow.

The Hand

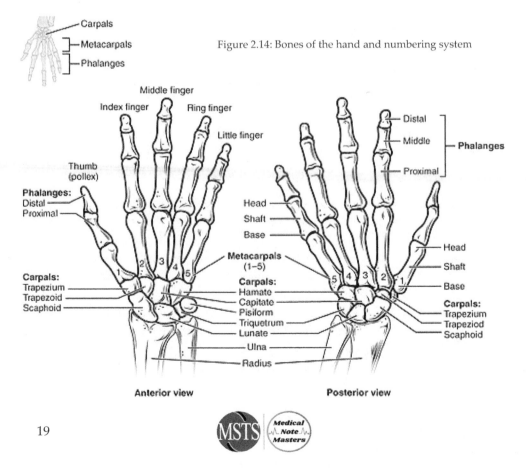

Figure 2.14: Bones of the hand and numbering system

The bones of the hand are essential landmarks for injuries that occur to the wrist, hand and fingers. The fingers may be described with layperson terms (like index, middle, ring, or pinky finger) or by more technical numbering in which the thumb is the 1st digit, and the pinky is the 5th digit.

- **Radius and Ulna** - the radius and ulna are the bones of the forearm that articulate with the carpal bones to form the wrist joint, with the radius on the thumb side and the ulna on the pinky side.

- **Carpals** – there are eight separate small carpal bones. The anatomic terms are infrequently used in the physical exam with one exception – the scaphoid – and the provider may specify that its overlying area is nontender. The anatomy of the scaphoid makes it susceptible to special injuries.

- **Metacarpals** – the bones in each digit that make up the body of the hand.

- **Phalanges** – the three individual bones in each finger (except for the thumb, which only has two bones). They are known as the proximal, middle, and distal phalanges (*singular phalanx*).

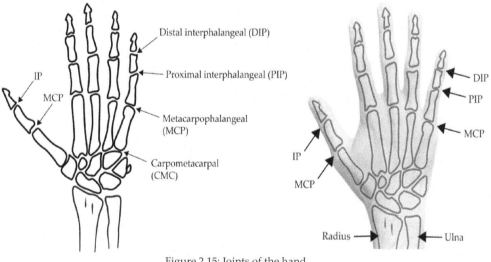

Figure 2.15: Joints of the hand

When describing injuries, the joints are more apparent external landmarks than bones and you will encounter these terms and abbreviations regularly.

- **Carpometacarpal (CMC) joint** – the joint created by the joining of the carpals to the metacarpals.

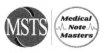

- **Metacarpophalangeal (MCP) joint** – the joint made by the connection of the metacarpals to the proximal phalanges. These joints form what are typically called the "knuckles."

- **Proximal interphalangeal (PIP) joint** – this is the first of two joints that are formed by the three phalanges in each finger. A laceration could be described as "just distal to the 2nd PIP joint," which would mean the patient has a laceration overlying the middle phalanx of the index finger.

- **Distal interphalangeal (DIP) joint** – this is the second of two joints formed by the three phalanges in each finger. Just like the PIP joint, the DIP joint is a common landmark when describing finger injuries.

- The thumb only has two phalanges so instead of having two separate joints (the PIP and DIP), it has one **interphalangeal (IP) joint.**

The Lower Body

- **Sacrum** – the fused bony region that connects the lumbar vertebrae to the coccyx (i.e. the tailbone, the small pointy structure at the bottom of the sacrum), and the two ilium hip "wing" bones to each other.

- **Pelvis** – the pelvis is the composite structure formed by the fusion of the sacrum and the two "hip" bones (that are actually made of three fused bones called the ilium, ischium, and pubis).

- **Femur** – the large bones that run the length of the thigh. The proximal portion articulates with the pelvis, and the distal portion articulates with the tibia. A "hip" fracture is the colloquial term for a proximal femur fracture, which typically occurs at the neck of the femur.

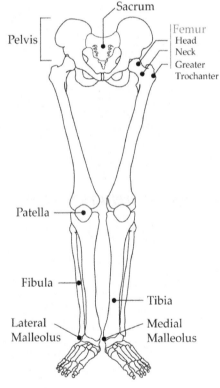

Figure 2.16: Bones and joints of the lower extremities

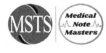

- o Femoral head – the "ball" that forms the ball and socket of the hip joint by connecting to the acetabulum (the "socket" in the ilium)
- o Femoral neck – the narrowed portion of the proximal femur connecting the femoral head to the greater trochanter, which is the most common area to sustain a "hip" fracture
- o Greater trochanter – the large, palpable bony protrusion on the lateral proximal femur

- **Patella** – the floating bone that is embedded in the patellar tendon and is commonly known as the kneecap.

- **Tibia** – the large "shin" bone in the medial lower leg that bears nearly all of the weight of the lower leg. It articulates with the femur to form the knee joint and to the foot to form the ankle joint.

- **Fibula** –smaller bone in the lateral lower leg that bears little weight.

- **Malleoli** – bony protrusions on the medial and lateral aspects of each ankle are formed by the ends of the tibia and fibula, respectively.

The major joints of the lower extremities include:

- **Hip joint** – a ball-and-socket joint formed by the femoral head "ball" and the cavity in the pelvis ("the socket") called the acetabulum. This joint is often replaced, and like the shoulder ball-and-socket joint, it can dislocate.

- **Knee joint** – the joint formed by the articulation of the femur and tibia. There are several soft tissues within the knee as pictured that are examined using ROM and specialized knee maneuvers since eliciting crepitus, pain or laxity can help localize internal soft tissue injuries.

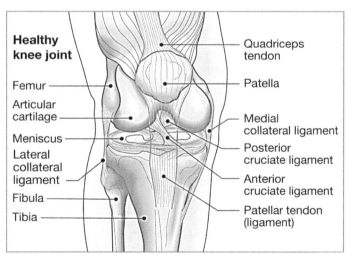

Figure 2.17: Schematic knee anatomy

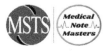

The Foot

The foot is organized in nearly the same fashion as the hand.

- **Tarsal bones** – the tarsal bones compose the body of the foot

- **Metatarsals** – the metatarsals compose the distal half of the foot, between the tarsal bones and toes, and have visible overlying tendons. The base of the fifth metatarsal is often involved in "rolling out" ankle injuries.

- **Phalanges** – the toes are nearly identical in structure to the fingers. Note that like the thumb, the big toe (or great toe) is only made up of two bones, rather than three bones (proximal, middle, distal) like the rest of the toes.

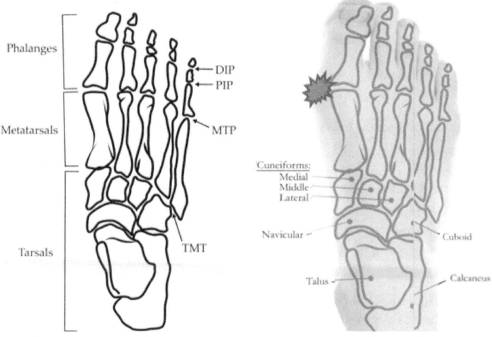

Figure 2.18: Bones and joints of the foot

The joints of the feet occur in the same general anatomic location as the joints of the hands and are named similarly. The **tarsometatarsal (TMT)** joint, **metatarsophalangeal (MTP)** joint, and the two **interphalangeal (proximal interphalangeal, distal interphalangeal)** joints are again significant landmarks for describing pain, swelling, redness, etc. that occur in the feet. For example, gout typically causes pain and redness in the 1st MTP joint (the "knuckle" of the big toe, marked with red callout in figure).

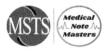

Female Anatomy

Internal Anatomy

Female internal anatomy is classically depicted in Figure 2.19. Although the scribe cannot see these structures, the physician will use these terms to describe the exam, radiology results, and other sections of documentation. Hence, the scribe needs to be familiar with these terms and spelling.

- Fundus – the "top" of the uterus, often measured during later pregnancy
- Ovary – small ovoid glands that produce female hormones and release eggs. They are prone to cysts and other maladies that can cause pain.
- Corpus luteum – the follicle that released a recently fertilized egg, sometimes develops a symptomatic cyst, seen on ultrasound.
- Endometrium – the innermost lining of the uterus, which cyclically grows and sheds during menses. It is also associated with endometriosis.
- Myometrium – the middle muscular portion of the uterus, which can contract and cramp. It is also the layer where fibroids most often occur.
- Fallopian tube – the tube leading to the uterus from the ovary, where egg and sperm travel, and where fertilization may occur.

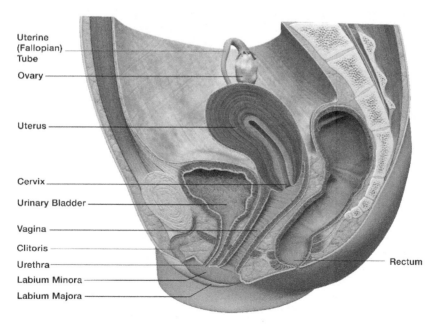

Figure 2.19: Internal female reproductive anatomy, sagittal view

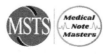

External Anatomy

While the term "vagina" is often colloquially used to refer to all of the female genitalia, it only refers to the canal that connects external anatomy to the cervical opening. The external female anatomy is called the vulva, which includes:

- Mons pubis – a layer of adipose that overlies the pubic symphysis.
- Labia majora – two folds of skin and adipose covered in pubic hair that cover and protect the inner vulvar structures.
- Labia minora – moist inner skin folds, lacking pubic hair, that reach from the clitoris to the vulva vestibule.
- Clitoris – a bulb-like collection of erectile tissue and nerves.
- Vulva vestibule – the area that lies between the labia minora that contains the vaginal orifice, the urethral orifice, and gland ducts.
- Orifices – the "openings" to an inner structure.
- Vulvar glands, such as Bartholin's – produce mucus to aid in lubrication, that may become clogged and infected.

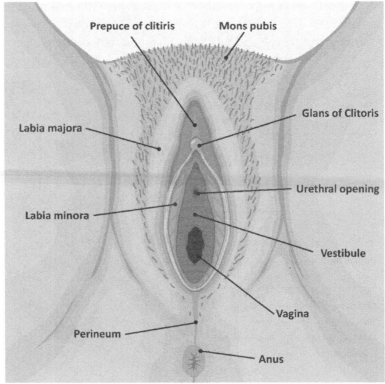

Figure 2.20: External female reproductive anatomy

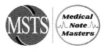

The Language of Medicine

As you work your way through this training, you will notice that many of the terms used are not in plain English. In fact, the medical terminology is so different from English that many consider it to be a foreign language that requires dedicated study. If you anticipate a medical career, learning the language now will have lifelong value. Reviewing these roots frequently alongside your medical documentation will help you absorb this new language, and over time, it will become second-nature.

Greek and Latin Root Words

Much of the English language is derived from Greek and Latin root words, but especially in medical terminology. You may likely notice that you have seen many of these roots in daily words, and studying them here increases base language skills that can be applied to standardized tests or learning a foreign language.

To reinforce your learning, consider using our online flashcard quiz here: https://quizlet.com/103142699. Online training that incorporates audio will help you more easily recognize terms as your provider says them.

Table 2.1: Greek and Latin root words – prefixes

Root	Definition	Example
A/n-	None, lacking, without	Apnea (not breathing), anoxia (lack of oxygen)
Ab-	Away from	Abduction (move away from)
Actin/o-	Light	Actinic keratosis (skin lesions from years of sun exposure)
Ad-	Toward	Adhesion (sticking to)
Adip/o-	Relating to fat	Adipose tissue (fat)
Angi/o-	Blood vessel	Angiogram (blood vessel imaging)
Ankyl(o)-	Stiff	Ankylosing spondylitis (a type of spinal arthritis)
Anter/o-	Front	Anterior (front side)
Arthr/o-	Joints	Arthritis (inflammation of the joints)
Ather/o-	Plaque	Atherosclerosis (hardening of the arteries)
Aur-	Ear	Auricle (visible portion of the ear)

Axilla/o-	Armpit	Axillary abscess (abscess in the armpit)
Balan/o-	Penis	Balantis (inflammation of the penis)
Bary-	Weight, pressure	Bariatric surgery (weight loss surgery)
Blephar/o-	Eyelid	Blepharoplasty (eyelid surgery)
Brady-	Slow	Bradycardia (slow heart rate)
Bronch-	Pulmonary tubes	Bronchitis (inflammation of the bronchi)
Bucc-	Cheek	Buccal (relating to the inside of the mouth, especially the cheek)
Burs/o-	Bursa (fluid-filled sacs near joints)	Bursitis (inflammation of the bursa)
Carcin/o-	Cancerous	Carcinoma (a category of cancer)
Cardi-	Heart	Electrocardiogram (record of the electricity of the heart)
Carp/o-	Carpals (wrist bones)	Carpal tunnel syndrome (compression of nerve in wrist)
Cervic/o-	Neck	Cervix (neck of the uterus)
Co/n-	Together, with	Coagulation (clot coming together)
Contra-	Against, opposite	Contraception (against conception)
Cost/o-	Rib	Costal cartilage (cartilage that connects a rib to the breastbone)
Cry/o-	Cold	Cryotherapy (using cold liquid to freeze and destroy abnormal skin cells)
Cutane/o	Skin	Subcutaneous (under the skin)
Cyt/o-	Cells	Cytology (examining cells)
Derm/o-	Skin	Dermatology (the study of the skin)
Diaphor/o-	Sweating	Diaphoretic (sweaty)
Dipl/o-	Double, two	Diplopia (double vision)
Dors/o-	Back (of body)	Dorsal (pertaining to the back or posterior of a structure)
Dys-	Abnormal	Dysuria (painful or difficult urination)
Ecto-	Out, outside	Ectopic pregnancy (a pregnancy outside the uterus)
Enter/o-	Intestines	Gastroenteritis (inflammation of the stomach and intestines)

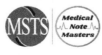

Epi-	Above, upon	Epiglottis (a thin valve-like structure that covers the glottis while swallowing)
Epitheli/o-	Skin	Epithelium (the cellular covering of internal and external surfaces of the body)
Erythem/o-	Flushed, redness	Erythematous (exhibiting abnormal redness of the skin)
Erythr/o-	Red	Erythrocyte (red blood cell)
Eu-	Good, normal	Euthyroid (normal thyroid function)
Ex-	Out, away from	Exophthalmos (bulging out of the eye)
Gastr/o-	Stomach	Gastroenterology (the specialty of diseases of the stomach and intestines)
Ger/o-	Old age	Gerontology (specialists for the elderly)
Gyne-	Female	Gynecomastia (female breasts in a male)
Hemi-	Half	Hemiplegia (paralysis of half the body)
Hem/o-	Blood	Hematemesis (vomiting blood)
Hepat/o-	Liver	Hepatitis (inflammation of the liver)
Hyper-	Above, excess	Hypertension (high blood pressure)
Hypo-	Below, deficient	Hypotension (low blood pressure)
Hyster-	Uterus	Hysterectomy (surgical removal of uterus)
Idi/o-	Unknown	Idiopathic (unknown cause)
Inguin-	Groin	Inguinal hernia (hernia in groin area)
Kal/i-	Potassium	Hyperkalemia (high potassium)
Laryng/o-	Larynx, voice box	Laryngospasm (sudden tight and sustained closure of the vocal cords)
Leuk/o-	White	Leukocytes (white blood cells)
Litho-	Stone	Lithotripsy (the process of breaking up kidney stones)
Lux/o-	To slide	Subluxation (an incomplete or partial dislocation)
Macro-	Large	Macrocytosis (a condition in which red blood cells are unusually large)
Mammo-	Breast	Mammogram (breast imaging)
Micro-	Small	Microcytosis (a condition in which red blood cells are unusually small)

Melan/o-	Black	Melanin (a class of pigments that account for the dark color of skin or hair)
My/o-	Muscle	Myalgia (muscle aches and pains)
Narc-	Numbness, stupor	Narcolepsy (a condition that involves sudden attacks of sleep)
Natr/o-	Sodium	Hyponatremia (low sodium)
Neo-	New	Neonatal (relating to newborns)
Nephr/o-	Kidney	Nephropathy (disease of the kidney)
Neuro-	Nerve	Neuralgia (nerve pain)
Onc/o-	Tumor	Oncogenic (giving rise to or relating to tumor formation)
Onych/o-	Nail (fingers or toes)	Onychomycosis (fungal nail infection)
Ortho-	Straight, correct	Orthopedics (correction of deformities)
Ost/o-	Bone	Osteonecrosis (bone death)
Ot/o-	Ear	Otalgia (ear pain)
Pan-	All, entire	Pandemic (a disease attacking all)
Para-	Next to, beside	Parathyroid (glands next to the thyroid)
Peri-	Around	Periumbilical (area around the umbilicus)
Poly-	Much, many	Polyuria (excessive urination)
Poster/o-	Back (of body), behind	Posterior (situated behind or at the back of)
Pulmo-	Lungs	Pulmonologist (specialist in lung disease)
Pseudo-	False or fake	Pseudocyesis (false pregnancy)
Radicul/o-	Nerve root	Radiculopathy (irritation or injury to a nerve root)
Retro-	Back, backward, behind	Retrograde amnesia (inability to recall memories before an injury)
Squam/o-	Scale, thin/flat	Squamous (consisting of scales)
Super-	Above, beyond	Superficial (top surface layer)
Supra-	Above, upper	Suprapubic (above the pubic arch)
Tachy-	Fast	Tachycardia (fast heart rate)
Viscer/o-	Internal organs	Visceral (relating to, situated in, or affecting the internal organs)

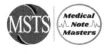

Table 2.2: Greek and Latin root words – suffixes

Root	Definition	Example
-algesia	Sensitivity to pain	Analgesia (pain relief)
-algia	Relating to pain	Myalgia (muscle aches and pains)
-arthria	Articulating words	Dysarthria (slurred, inarticulate speech)
-chezia	Defecation	Hematochezia (bloody stools)
-ectomy	Removal, excision	Hysterectomy (removal of the uterus)
-edema	Swelling	Lymphedema (fluid retention caused by a compromised lymphatic system)
-emia	Blood condition	Anemia (a lack of blood)
-esthesia	Feeling, sensibility	Paresthesia (an abnormal spontaneous sensation, like itching)
-gram or -graphy	Measure or image	Electrocardiogram (recording of the heart electrical activity)
-itis	Inflammation	Sinusitis (inflammation of the sinuses)
-mania	Madness	Kleptomania (impulsive stealing)
-ostomy	Opening	Colostomy (opening the colon to the skin)
-otomy	Incision, cut into	Craniotomy (surgery into the skull)
-oxia	Relating to oxygen	Hypoxia (low oxygen)
-paresis	Weakness, partial paralysis	Gastroparesis (weakened muscular contractions of the stomach)
-pareunia	Sexual intercourse	Dyspareunia (pain with intercourse)
-pathy	Dysfunction, disease	Neuropathy (dysfunction of a nerve)
-phagia	Eating, swallowing	Dysphagia (difficulty swallowing)
-pnea	Relating to breathing	Dyspnea (difficulty breathing)
-rrhage	Excessive flow	Hemorrhage (bleeding)
-rrhea	Flow	Rhinorrhea (runny nose)
-sclerosis	Hardening	Atherosclerosis (hardening of plaque)
-stasis	Lack of movement	Hemostasis (arrest of bleeding)
-staxis	Dripping	Epistaxis (nosebleed)
-stenosis	Narrowing, stricture	Spinal stenosis (narrowing spinal canal)
-tomy	Incision	Lobotomy (operation on the frontal lobe)
-trophy	To nourish	Atrophy (wasting away of body tissues)

Common Abbreviations

Because healthcare is a fast-paced industry, for years staff members used abbreviations to document frequently used terms. However, over time it became more evident that abbreviations can lead to miscommunication and medical errors, so now regulatory bodies have strong recommendations against most abbreviations. Nonetheless, many of the abbreviations shown may be present in older notes and are in common practice for non-official note-taking, so recognizing them is beneficial. You should not, as a rule, get into the habit of using abbreviations in medical documentation however.

Table 2.2: Common abbreviations and their meanings

ABx	antibiotics	EtOH	alcohol
A&O	alert and oriented	F/C	fever/chills
ASA	aspirin	Fx	fracture
BID	twice daily	G_P_	gravida para (pregnancy)
BM	bowel movement	HA	headache
BMP	Basic metabolic profile	f/u	Follow-up
BS	bowel sounds or blood sugar	h/o	History of
CBC	Complete blood count	Hx	history
C&S	Culture & sensitivity	Bx	Biopsy
C/C/E	Cyanosis/clubbing/edema	IM	intramuscular
C/o	complains of	IV	intravenous
CP	chest pain	IVF	IV fluids
CTA	clear to auscultation	JVD	jugular venous distention
C/w	consistent with	LAD	lymphadenopathy
CXR	Chest Xray	LMP	Last menstrual period
D/C	Discharge or discontinue	LOC	Loss/level of consciousness
DM	Diabetes mellitus	MOI	mechanism of injury
Ddx	differential diagnosis	MVA/ MVC	motor vehicle accident or collision
D/T	due to	ROM	range of motion
Dx	diagnosis	RRR	regular rate and rhythm

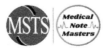

EBL	estimated blood loss (from surgery)	NAD	no acute disease/ no acute distress (contextual)
EMS	emergency medical service	SL	sublingual (under tongue)
NT ND	Nontender nondistended	S/P	status post (surgical)
NPO	nothing by mouth	Sx	symptoms
NS	normal saline	SOB	shortness of breath
N/V	nausea/vomiting	TID	three times daily
PERRL	pupils equal, round and reactive to light	TM	tympanic membrane
PO	per os (orally)	TTP	tenderness to palpation
URI	Upper respiratory infection	UTD	up-to-date
PRN	as needed	VSS	vital signs stable
PTA	prior to arrival / admission	WNL	within normal limits
QD	Daily	QID	Four times daily
QHS	Nightly/bedtime	Y/o	year old

End of Chapter Quiz

1. Which term best describes the location of the big toe on the foot?
    a. Medial
    b. Lateral
    c. Proximal
    d. Ventral

2. Palms of the hand and soles of the feet can be described by which term?
    a. Distal
    b. Dorsal
    c. Volar
    d. Posterior

3. The belly button is more technically known by which term?
    a. Epigastric region
    b. Pubis
    c. Periumbilical region
    d. Umbilicus

4. True or False: the knee is distal to the foot.
    a. True
    b. False

5. True or False: the thumb is located on the ulnar aspect of the hand.
    a. True
    b. False

6. The back of the head is more technically known as which part of the scalp?
    a. Occipital
    b. Temporal
    c. Parietal
    d. Frontal

7. Which description below best describes the location of a fingerprint?
    a. Proximal volar phalanx
    b. Proximal dorsal phalanx
    c. Distal volar phalanx
    d. Distal plantar phalanx

8. The ribs connect to the sternum via which anatomical structure?

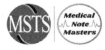

a. AC joint

b. Costal cartilage

c. Malleoli

d. Interphalangeal joint

9. Which term is NOT an anterior landmark?

a. Acromioclavicular joint

b. Sternum

c. Clavicles

d. Costovertebral angle

10. The term -sclerosis refers to softening

a. True

b. False

11. Which term describes low central abdominal pain?

a. Suprapubic

b. Umbilical

c. Supraumbilical

d. Periumbilical

12. Which root word refers to the liver?

a. Cardio-

b. Nephro-

c. Hepato-

d. Dermato-

13. What is the medical term for the "groin" area?

a. Suprapubic

b. Periumbilical

c. Inguinal

d. Femoral

14. The abbreviation "prn" means "as needed."

a. True

b. False

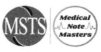

3. The Subjective Sections

The primary responsibility of the medical scribe is to create the medical note based on what is observed and heard during the patient visit. Most scribes will type this note in real-time into the EHR on a laptop, as the provider is interviewing and

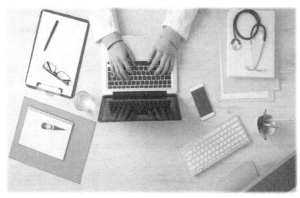

examining the patient. In other situations, the scribe may hand-write notes on a clipboard in the patient's room, and then transfer them into the EHR immediately afterward.

You will first learn the structure of the medical note in its purest form before seeing it used in practice. The EHR will significantly influence how the information is entered and formatted but there are far too many variations to cover EHR training here. Most facilities have a brief EHR training course for new employees so you will learn those specifics later.

The Golden Rules

If the doctor discusses it, document it.

While observing a patient visit, certain items discussed may seem extraneous or irrelevant, and it may be tempting to omit things that don't appear necessary on the surface. Do not fall into that trap! Typically, a provider on a tight schedule does not waste time on questions that do not have a purpose, so even if the question seems irrelevant to you, it should still be documented. Similarly, the physician may explain lab results or the treatment plan to the patient in layman's terms that may not seem like something "official" to put in the note, but a good scribe knows to document that plan in medical terms.

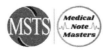

If it isn't documented, it didn't happen.

When providers or other parties look back upon a note, it cannot be assumed that something occurred unless it was written down. The typical error here is again omitting things that are routine or assumed. We all know what happens with assumptions right? Unfortunately, something that seems obvious at the time of the visit does not come across in the note, and someone reading it later misses out. During an exam it may be obvious that a patient is demented, intoxicated or agitated, but if you do not document that the history is limited and provide a description, then the record indicates the patient was unimpaired. A physician may be in the habit of "always" performing a heart and lung exam, but if it is not documented, then later on, the physician cannot definitively say that particular patient had the exam performed. Essentially, someone reading the note later should be able to get a sense of the whole picture of the visit.

SOAP Note

The general form of almost all medical notes is the "SOAP" format, which stands for Subjective, Objective, Assessment, and Plan. In some cases, providers rearrange to an "APSO" note to prioritize the Assessment and Plan, which is discussed in Chapter 5. These sections correspond to the general order of information within most medical notes and are summarized below.

Subjective: The subjective section is based on information the patient tells the provider—since it is relayed from the patient's personal perspective, it is deemed "subjective." The chief complaint, history of present illness, and review of systems fall into this category. The past medical history, social history, medications, allergies, and family history also fall under this category when this information is obtained from the patient or similar sources.

Objective: The objective section is based on information obtained by the physician and the healthcare team, who are deemed objective, unbiased evaluators of the patient. This section includes vital signs, physical exam, labs, radiology results, and any other data collected during the visit.

Assessment: Based on the subjective and objective pieces of information, the provider makes an assessment. This section outlines the diagnoses and the

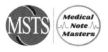

physician's thought process about the case, called "Clinical Decision Making" or "Medical Decision Making."

Plan: Given the diagnosis, the treatment plan describes any future orders like labs, imaging studies, referrals, or changes to the patient's prescription and over-the-counter medications. Lastly, the plan will suggest a timeframe for follow-up.

General Medical Note Outline

The medical note is often constructed in the order below, and we will break down each section in greater detail in the following chapters.

Subjective:

Chief Complaint (CC) i.e. Reason for Visit (RFV)
History of Present Illness (HPI)
Review of Systems (ROS)
Allergies
Medications
Past Medical History (PMHx)
Past Surgical History (PSHx)
Family History (FHx)
Social History (SHx)

Objective:

Physical Exam (PE)
Laboratory Results
Imaging Results
Clinical Course/Re-evaluations
Consultations

Assessment:

Clinical Decision Making/Medical Decision Making (MDM)
Diagnoses

Plan:

Discharge Medications
Patient Instructions
Work or school notes
Referrals and follow-up

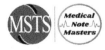

Chief Complaint (CC)/Reason for Visit (RFV)

The chief complaint is simply a brief one or a few-word phrase stating why the patient presented for medical evaluation. Another term for this is Reason for Visit, which reflects that a patient does not always have a "complaint." In many cases, clinical staff will enter a chief complaint into the EHR during the intake process, so the physician has an idea in advance of what the patient's primary concern is. Unfortunately, most EHRs require a single selection from a prepopulated pick-list, which may not include an exact match for what the patient said. Hence, the physician typically confirms this information. Most EHRs also pull this information into the note automatically, so the scribe may have to make manual clarification if the CC reported to staff is not truly the reason for the visit. Some providers may begin the visit with a phrase such as, "So I see you're here for X, is that right?"

Common examples of CCs include chest pain, cough, or abdominal pain. Because the chief complaint is part of the subjective section, it should be a complaint stated by the patient, and not a diagnosis. For example, abdominal pain is an appropriate chief complaint, but appendicitis—even if the patient believes that's what it is—is not a chief complaint. However, when patients do already have an established diagnosis and are coming in for a follow-up, the Reason for Visit might be "Follow up Diabetes" for example. Below are some other common RFVs, which will vary substantially depending on the type of clinical setting.

Table 3.1: Common chief complaints/reasons for visit

Abdominal pain	Diabetic check	Shortness of breath
Back pain	URI/Cough	Vaginal bleeding
Headache	Rash	Medication refill
SOB/Asthma	Pregnancy check	ER f/u
Sore throat	Vomiting	Chest pain
Fatigue	Fever	Motor vehicle accident
Ankle sprain	Knee pain, shoulder pain	Work note
Ear pain	Dysuria	Annual physical
BP check	Dizziness	Anxiety
Altered mental status	Psychiatric evaluation	Laceration
Seizure	Pre-op assessment	Immunizations

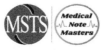

History of Present Illness (HPI)

The HPI follows the chief complaint, and it is a concise narrative of the patient's story, given by the patient but reorganized by the scribe. You will derive the necessary information for the HPI from the previous notes, the questions asked by the provider, and the answers given by the patient, family, or others. Although there is no official right or wrong way to write the HPI, medical providers have been using a relatively standard format for many years, and deviating from that format makes the HPI more difficult for providers to interpret. Distilling the patient information chronologically and in order of priority will take time to learn, but it is a skill that will serve you well throughout your medical career.

A patient seldom provides the history in the format needed for the HPI, so you must learn to reorganize and synthesize the information into a more coherent narrative. Because of the pace with which many providers ask questions, you will usually need to develop a shorthand so you can keep up with the conversation without missing important information. Using a one-page template with the note elements and other reminders outlined also assists with quicker note-taking.

We will soon detail the standard structure of the HPI, but to give you a sense of the final product, here is a sample HPI for a diabetic follow-up visit:

> *John Smith is a 55-year-old male with a history of hypertension and poorly controlled type II diabetes who presents for a diabetic check. He was last seen three months ago, at which time his A1c was 10.3, and he was started on Lantus 10 units at night in addition to his prior regimen of glipizide ER 10 mg and metformin 750 mg BID. Since then, he has been feeling well without any weight changes, visual changes, lower extremity paresthesias, polyuria, or polyphagia. His morning blood sugars are typically around 150 and up to 180 after eating. He denies any episodes of symptomatic hypoglycemia.*

Let's now go through the HPI step-by-step.

Step 0: Check for Background Info

For established patients and especially those presenting with an RFV of *Follow Up X Condition*, the prepared scribe will first reference prior notes and collect information in the EHR that is pertinent to today's visit. Based on the clinic schedule, the scribe can utilize any downtime by looking up information on future patients and being

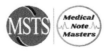

prepared with a brief summary of the background to the visit. Great scribes don't just wait for data to come – they go and find it! Being able to bring this information to the provider in advance of entering the patient's room can significantly streamline visits, and you will document this information into the HPI in a later step.

Step 1: Source of Information

Upon starting the patient visit, take a quick assessment of who is providing the history. In most cases, it is presumed that the patient is the primary, reliable source of information. However, in many cases, the HPI comes from other sources, such as family members, nursing home staff, or an ambulance crew. The source of information is typically documented at the very beginning of the HPI, and most EHRs have a designated area for this documentation. If there is no discrete EHR area, the scribe can manually enter this information before the HPI body as a stand-alone line. For example:

> *History was obtained from the patient and husband through a Spanish interpreter.*

Any limitations to obtaining a complete history should also be noted, such as, "History is limited by patient intoxication." Alternatively, the clinician may indicate that "the patient is deemed a reliable historian," but using this phrase is less common because it is assumed that the patient is a reasonably reliable historian. In any case, the scribe should document source(s) and limitations to the history, since this information can be quite valuable from a medicolegal perspective if the reliability or accuracy of the HPI is ever called into question.

Step 2: The First Topic Sentence

Typically, the first sentence of an HPI includes the patient's name, age, sex*, a brief mention of pertinent medical history, and then the chief complaint. It should provide just enough information to act as a topic sentence without being too long or wordy. The basic format is:

> *Name* is a(n) *age* y.o. *sex** with a history of *past medical history* who presents with *chief complaint*…

> *John Doe* is a *23-year-old male* with a history of *asthma* who presents with *shortness of breath*...

Often the EHR can pull in the name, age, and sex from the demographic information entered during registration, which is helpful to avoid spelling errors.

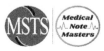

*This format has been in place for many years and traditionally specifies male or female, and you may even see race referenced as well. More recently, sexual identity is addressed with expanded terminology, and the EHR usually allows for non-binary sexual terms during registration including legal sex, sex assigned at birth, preferred names and preferred pronouns. If you are unsure what to write, stick with a generic term such as "the patient" rather than "him" or "her."

Step 3: The Backdrop Sentence

Most commonly, when the story permits, HPIs are written in a chronological order beginning with the oldest directly relevant information and working towards the present time.

According to this style, after the topic sentence, the HPI will mention any directly-related medical history to provide more background if needed. This may be a sentence or two that describes a recent ER visit, a recent exacerbation of epilepsy, etc. For example, if a patient was recently hospitalized and is presenting with shortness of breath, you would have looked up the recent notes in Step 0 to be briefly summarized in the second sentence. The first two sentences may appear like this:

> *Jane Doe is a 61-year-old female with a history of COPD who presents with shortness of breath. She was admitted from 7/1 to 7/3 for an acute exacerbation of COPD and discharged on tapered prednisone and Combivent...*

Providing this summary of any recent and directly-related healthcare encounters early in the HPI updates the reader on the patient's baseline medical status leading up to the present issue. This backdrop sentence is especially important for follow-up visits. In these cases, the second sentence summarizes the previous visit and any testing that has been performed in the interim. The sentences to follow will then describe how the patient has been doing since that last visit, as noted by the transition phrase "since then..."

For example:

> *John Doe is a 54-year-old male with a history of hypertension who presents with dizziness. His dose of metoprolol was increased from 50 mg BID to 100 mg BID on 8/15 and since then...*

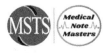

Josephina Thomas is a 62-year-old F with a history of CAD who presents for a medication check. The cardiologist recently started her on Lasix, and she was told to follow-up with primary care. Since starting Lasix, she has...

Laura Jimenez is a healthy 19 y/o F seen in the ER on 9/30 for a cat bite who presents for a wound check. No sutures were placed, and she was given a prescription for Augmentin. Since her ER visit, her wound has been...

The benefit of writing in this chronological style is that the HPI flows like a story, which makes it easier for you and future readers to follow and remember. Often, symptoms change and evolve, making it critical to outline the timing clearly.

Adam Smith is a 43-year-old male with a history of chronic back pain who presents with acute left low back pain. He was at his baseline, taking 1 Norco TID, until yesterday afternoon when he "tweaked" his back while lifting firewood.

Levi Jones is a 70 y/o M with a history of migraines who presents for headache. He typically takes propranolol as a preventative and seldom needs other medications, but now in the last 2 weeks he has had steadily increasing pain and went to the ER last night.

Usually, the most challenging part about writing the body of the HPI is that the patient rarely outlines symptoms in chronological order. This means that no matter how disorganized the history is told, you will need to make sense of it in the HPI. Many people mistakenly believe that scribes are like court stenographers, typing hundreds of words per minute, never missing a single one. However, a medical scribe is not just transcribing conversation word-for-word from one medium to the next but is reorganizing this information and writing it more concisely, accurately, and eloquently than it was relayed.

Step 4: The Body of the HPI and OPQRST

While you are writing the "body" of the HPI, the OPQRST mnemonic can help further clarify the patient's symptoms and summarize these essential details. OPQRST stands for Onset, Palliation/Provocation, Quality, Region/Radiation, Severity, and Timing. Each of these letters describes something about the patient's symptoms, as explained below.

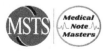

Onset—onset describes the time of onset of the patient's symptoms. In our last examples, the beginning of his back pain was yesterday afternoon, and the headaches started getting worse two weeks ago. That is the most straightforward definition of "onset," but it can also be helpful to describe the context in which symptoms arose, such as:

"The headache began suddenly two days ago while eating dinner."

Palliative and Provocative — palliative refers to what makes the patient's symptoms better, and provocative refers to what causes the symptoms to worsen. For example, in a patient with leg pain, is it worse while bearing weight? Is it better while elevated? Sometimes nothing makes the patient's pain better or worse, which is documented as well.

Quality—quality describes the patient's symptoms with more adjectives and descriptions. The provider may ask, "What does it feel like?" but sometimes patients in pain have some difficulty finding the words. Usually referring to pain, patients may describe it as sharp, dull, burning, pins/needles, pressure-like, etc., or describe it as being similar to the pain they've had before. For example:

"Doc, this feels like I'm getting stabbed, just like the time I had that kidney stone."

Region/Radiation—region describes the primary location of pain, and radiation describes any secondary areas that it seems to involve. Pain may seem to be primarily in one place and move into another place, which is called radiation. An example is in chest pain, where the pain is mainly in the chest but may radiate into the neck or arm, or low back pain that radiates down the leg. Pain can be described as localized or non-radiating if contained in a defined area.

Severity – severity describes how intense the symptom is. For example, a patient's pain may be rated as 10/10. In some cases, the patient may describe the severity of pain in words like mild, moderate, or severe (or any number of synonyms), and these too would be descriptors of severity.

Timing—timing refers to how the symptoms change over time. Fundamentally, symptoms are either constant (always present) or intermittent (come and go) and can also be described with words like suddenly, gradually, progressively, waxing/waning, building up, etc. Some people also consider a history of similar symptoms to belong in Timing as well, such as:

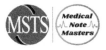

"Doc, this feels just like the time I had that kidney stone."
or
"I've never had anything like this before."

Some add an "A" onto the end of the OPQRST mnemonic for Associated symptoms (i.e., OPQRSTA), although it doesn't follow the alphabetic order. Associated symptoms refers to additional symptoms that the patient may have in addition to the primary symptom. For instance, in a person with abdominal pain, the physician will often ask if there is Associated nausea.

Even though the OPQRST system may seem like too much to include in the HPI, it does not mean that the HPI can't be written concisely. Usually, you can include several OPQRST details in a single sentence. For example: "...pain is sharp, located over the epigastrium, and worse after eating." Just remember, if the doctor discussed it, you should document it!

The HPI for our previous patient following up for hypertension would look like this:

> *"John Doe is a 54-year-old male with a history of hypertension who presents for a medication check and dizziness. His dose of metoprolol was increased from 50 mg BID to 100 mg BID on 8/15 (O), and since then (O), he has been light-headed intermittently (T). It usually happens when going from a seated to standing position (P) and improves when lying down (P). It is worst first thing in the morning and yesterday morning (T) it was 'really bad' (S), and he nearly fell walking to the bathroom. He describes it as feeling faint (Q), not a spinning sensation (Q). No lower extremity swelling, changes in urine output, or palpitations (A)."*

Step 5: Wrapping up the HPI

The remainder of the HPI is a catch-all of other supplemental history and pertinent negatives. In the most straightforward cases, this may include writing "no history of similar symptoms." More complex patients may need an additional paragraph to include other symptoms, side issues, or further information about the patient's past medical history (or lack thereof). If you follow the *Golden Rule of scribing—if the provider discusses it, document it—* then you will know to collect miscellaneous information and pertinent negatives. For instance, our patient John Doe might wrap up like this:

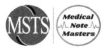

He denies a history of similar symptoms. No history of stroke. No vision changes, nausea, vomiting. No recent travel. He also states he is pretty frustrated with how many different medications he is on for HTN and would like to know if some of his meds can be discontinued.

Changing a Patient's Words into Medical Terminology

One way to reduce the number of words required in a note is to use medical terms for a patient's symptoms. Patients typically have no medical background and may need to use many words to try to describe something that can be documented more concisely with a medical term. Over time, these medical terms will become second nature to you and can save time during documentation. However, you must take care to use the word accurately such that the term doesn't draw a conclusion. Some examples are shown below, but if no medical term exists, you can simply use the patient's wording in quotes. The Review of Systems, discussed next, is a comprehensive list of questions used to survey patients about various symptoms, and using medical terminology can save space and time. Using medical terms in the subjective sections is good practice to learn terminology, but is not necessary.

Table 3.2: Patient's words to medical terminology

Medical Term	Definition/Example
Phonophobia	Sensitivity to sound. *"Any kind of noise is horrible, like extra loud."*
Photophobia	Sensitivity to light. *"The light really hurts my eyes. I had to stay inside."*
Sputum	Mucus that has been expelled during a cough. *"I was hacking up all kinds of green and yellow junk."*
Urinary frequency	Frequent urination. *"I had to go pee like a million times yesterday."*
Syncope	Loss of consciousness and postural tone, to "pass out" or "faint." If, in fact, the patient had a seizure, using the term syncope would be misleading.

Some EHRs utilize click box templates for HPI and/or ROS entry, designed in hopes of saving time during documentation, and also for billing purposes as discussed later. These templates are built only for common chief complaints, such as headache pictured in the figure, and some providers may prefer these for quick, low-risk visits.

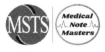

HPI Headache

HPI: Headache

CONCERN [headache]

Onset [3 Week(s) ago ▼] Duration [3 Hour(s) ▼]   Severity [moderate ▼] Status ○ improved ○ no change ○ worse ● resolved

CL | 1 | 2 | 3 | 4 | 5 | 6 | 7 | 8 | 9 | 0 | .   CL | 1 | 2 | 3 | 4 | 5 | 6 | 7 | 8 | 9 | 10

Min(s) | Hr(s) | Day(s) | Wk(s) | Mo(s) | Yr(s)   Frequency ● intermittent ○ constant ○ daily ○ weekly ○ monthly

Location	Radiation	Quality	Timing
☐ entire head	☐ no		☐ daytime
☐ frontal left ☑ frontal right	☐ anterior	☐ binding ☐ pressure ☐ superficial	☐ menstrual periods
☐ ocular left ☐ ocular right	☐ posterior	☐ debilitating ☑ sharp ☐ throbbing	☐ upon awakening
☐ parietal left ☐ parietal right	☑ neck	☐ dull ☑ squeezing ☐ worst ever	☐ weekday
☐ temporal left ☐ temporal right	☐ shoulders	☐ lancinating ☐ stabbing	☐ weekend
☐ occipital ☐ vertex	☐ upper thorax		Other
Other	Other	Other	

Aggravated by	☐ nothing	Relieved by	☐ nothing	Context
☐ allergies ☐ head position		☐ analgesics		☐ recent head trauma
☐ anxiety ☐ foods		☐ bath ☐ ice ☐ prescription drugs		☐ recent MVA
☑ bright lights ☐ noise ☐ valsalva		☑ dark ☐ massage ☐ relaxation		
☐ caffeine ☑ stress ☐ weather		☐ decongestants ☐ OTC meds ☑ sleep		Other
☐ exercise Other		☐ distraction ☐ position ☐ stretching		
		☐ heat Other		

Associated Symptoms / Pertinent Negatives

Yes No		Yes No		Yes No		Yes No		
☑ ☐ blurred vision		☐ ☐ hemianopsia left		☐ ☐ personality change		☐ ☐ URI sxs		☐ No associated symptoms
☐ ☐ clear sinus discharge		☐ ☐ hemianopsia right		☐ ☐ phonophobia		☐ ☐ vision loss left		☐ No pertinent negatives
☐ ☐ dizziness		☐ ☐ LOC		☐ ☐ photophobia		☐ ☐ vision loss right		☐ All others negative
☐ ☐ double vision		☐ ☐ memory loss		☐ ☐ scintillations		☐ ☐ visual aura		Other associated symptoms
☐ ☐ family Hx migraine		☑ ☐ nausea		☐ ☐ scotomata		☐ ☐ vertigo		
☐ ☐ fever		☐ ☐ neurological symptoms		☐ ☐ stiff neck		☐ ☐ vomiting		Other pertinent negatives
☐ ☐ head trauma		☑ ☐ performance changes						

Comments ☐ childhood motion sickness ☐ history of migraines ☐ ice cream headache ☐ sleepwalking

[OK]   [Cancel]

Figure 3.1: Example of click-box HPI entry in an EHR

Review of Systems (ROS)

The Review of Systems is ancillary history that is obtained either during or after the HPI. The intention is for the provider to systematically review all the body systems for other symptoms that were not volunteered in the HPI or may be more in the background, unrelated to the RFV. You could think of it in the context of the physician covering the HPI then asking, "Is there anything else going on?" For an acute visit, the ROS is not usually a priority because the provider is focused on the presenting complaint. For a yearly physical, however, these background symptoms might be more important to ensure a thorough evaluation, so the provider and staff may spend more time screening for background symptoms. At times, the patient is presented with a screening questionnaire to fill out in the waiting room to cover the common questions of an ROS, or intake personnel may review common questions.

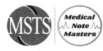

Documenting symptom elements in the review of systems is optimal for billing and coding reasons that changed in 2021 for outpatient clinics only, but remains unchanged for the emergency room and inpatient (see Chapter 7). In previous years, the billing level of the visit was partially determined by counting ROS elements, so providers made sure to include a thorough ROS. It is likely that clinic providers will continue to document a brief ROS after 2021 because they are accustomed to covering the ROS in the note and the ROS is included in existing note templates.

Questions for the review of systems are often phrased as a quick list of possible symptoms and may sound something like this:

> *"OK, so aside from this bad back pain, have you had other symptoms troubling you? Any spotting, belly pain, bowel problems, weight changes?"*

The ROS is completed more like a checklist—either a patient has the symptom on that list, or they do not. For the example above, the ROS might look like the list below. Alternatively, providers may prefer terms like "denies" or "no," or the EHR may have pos/neg checkboxes.

> *General: NEGATIVE weight changes*
> *GI: NEGATIVE bowel problems*
> *GU: NEGATIVE vaginal bleeding*
> *Musculoskeletal: POSITIVE LBP, per HPI*

There is no further description of positive findings (like sharp, radiating, etc.) but simply the presence or absence of it, since any positive symptoms need to be addressed in more detail in the HPI. Your provider may elect to write only "per HPI" for the ROS sections covered by the HPI, rather than duplicating the symptoms as positive or negative in the ROS. This practice saves time, but the more detailed ROS documentation is more valuable for your learning process by gaining practice associating symptoms to different body systems and using medical terminology to describe symptoms.

Many scribes initially struggle with differentiating the review of systems from the physical exam, because they both list body systems in a similar format. It may help you to think of the ROS as the "review of symptoms" because ROS includes only symptoms verbally mentioned by the patient; remember, it is included in the Subjective section of the medical note and therefore is based on information provided by the patient. The physical exam, in contrast, is part of the Objective section and includes the provider's observations of the patient, excluding symptoms.

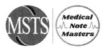

Given the 2021 billing guidelines, it is unlikely that the provider will spend a lot of time asking numerous questions to cover a full 14-system ROS. However, clinics who have found symptom review useful in the form of a questionnaire or intake screening may continue to include ROS in some form. The following tables list symptoms often covered in the ROS for reinforcement regarding using medical terms, not because you are likely to hear a provider ask about all of these symptoms.

1. Constitutional System

The constitutional system refers to symptoms that are general or widespread.

Medical Term	Definition
Changes in weight	Weight gain or loss, preferably specified in pounds/kilos
Chills	Sense of feeling cold and shivering
Fatigue	Feeling unusually tired, decreased energy
Fever	Measured temperature above 100.4°F or 38°C. If not measured, but the patient feels warm as though feverish, then referred to as "subjective" fever
Malaise	Feeling generally unwell
Myalgias	Muscle or body aches ("myo" referring to muscle and "algia" referring to pain)
Night sweats	Sweating at night while resting or asleep, not associated with exercise or heat
Diaphoresis	Sweating not associated with usual triggers

2. Eyes

Medical Term	Definition
Watery eyes	Excessive production of tears
Discharge	Fluid or pus drainage from the eye
Diplopia	Double vision ("Di" = two or split, and "–plopia" referring to vision)
Blurry vision	Self-explanatory
Photophobia	Excess sensitivity to light

3a. Ears (Combined in the ENT system)

Medical Term	Definition
Hearing loss	Difficulty hearing speech or other sounds

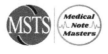

Otalgia	Ear pain ("oto" refers to the ears and "algia" refers to pain)
Otorrhea	Ear discharge ("oto" refers to the ears and "-rrhea" means discharge/drainage)
Tinnitus	Ear ringing. Pronounced "TIN-ni-tus" or "tin-NYE-tus"

3b. Nose (usually combined in the ENT system)

Medical Term	Definition
Congestion	Presence of thick nasal mucus
Epistaxis	Bloody nose
Rhinorrhea	Runny nose ("rhino" refers to the nose and "-rrhea" means drainage/discharge)

3c. Throat (usually combined in the ENT system)

Medical Term	Definition
Dysphagia	Difficulty swallowing ("dys" meaning abnormal and "phagia" referring to the act of swallowing)
Hoarseness	A raspy or strained voice
Snoring	Loud, snorting or grunting sounds made while sleeping

4. Cardiovascular

Medical Term	Definition
Chest pain	Any type of pain over the anterior thorax
Lower extremity edema	Swelling (edema) typically in association with heart failure or poor venous blood flow
Orthopnea	Shortness of breath while lying down ("ortho" means straight and "-pnea" refers to breathing)
Palpitations	A subjective sense that a person's heartbeat is abnormal; a patient may describe his/her heart rate as fast, pounding, slow, irregular, skipping, etc.

5. Respiratory

Medical Term	Definition
Cough	To suddenly expel air from the lungs with audible noise

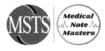

Dyspnea	Difficulty breathing ("dys" means abnormal and "-pnea" refers to breathing)
Shortness of breath	Difficulty breathing
Sputum	Mucus expectorated from the mouth during a cough
Wheezing	A high-pitched whistling sound heard while breathing, typically during exhalation

6. Gastrointestinal

Medical Term	Definition
Abdominal pain	Pain located anywhere in the abdominal region
Constipation	Infrequent or hard bowel movements (BMs)
Diarrhea	Loose or watery bowel movements (BMs)
Dysphagia	Difficulty swallowing
Hematochezia	Bright red blood passed rectally (BRBPR)
Melena	Dark, tarry, or coffee-ground stools
Nausea	The sensation that one might vomit
Vomiting	To eject stomach contents through the mouth

7a. Genitourinary

Medical Term	Definition
Dysuria	Painful urination often described as burning
Erectile dysfunction	Inability to develop or maintain an erection
Hematuria	Blood in the urine
Nocturia	The necessity to urinate during the night/sleep
Oliguria	Decreased urine output
Polyuria	Increased urine output
Urinary frequency	Urinating frequently, not necessarily related to volume
Urinary incontinence	Loss of bladder control
Urinary retention	Inability to empty the bladder fully
Urinary urgency	The sensation that one has to urinate urgently

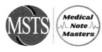

7b. Genitourinary (female organ-specific)

Medical Term	Definition
Dysmenorrhea	Painful menstrual periods
Dyspareunia	Pain with sexual intercourse
Irregular menses	Abnormal timing of menstrual periods
Menorrhagia	Heavy or prolonged periods
Menopause	Cessation of menses
Vaginal bleeding	Bleeding from the vagina, usually of uterine source
Vaginal discharge	Abnormal fluid from the vagina

8. Musculoskeletal

Medical Term	Definition
Arthralgia	Pain involving a joint (ankle, knee, elbow, shoulder, etc.)
Joint stiffness	Rigidity; moving with difficulty
Spasm	A sudden, involuntary muscle contraction
Swelling	Enlargement of body tissues, sometimes called "edema"

9. Integumentary (Skin or Dermatologic)

Medical Term	Definition
Laceration	Cut of the skin or tissues
Lesion	An abnormality of the skin
Pruritus	Itching or itchiness
Rash	Redness or irritation of the skin

10. Neurologic

Medical Term	Definition
Altered mental status (AMS)	A broadly applicable term including confusion and changes in memory
Paralysis	Loss of motor function
Paresis	Reduced motor function or strength
Paresthesia	Numbness, tingling, or burning sensation
Numbness	Loss of sensation

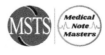

Seizures	Abnormal brain activity resulting in convulsive movements or changes in mental processes
Syncope	Loss of consciousness and postural tone, to "faint," pronounced "sink-o-pee"
Tremors	Involuntary shaking or quivering movements
Vertigo	Dizziness described as a spinning sensation; different than light-headedness
Weakness	Lacking usual motor strength

11. Psychiatric

Medical Term	Definition
Anxiety	Excessive unease or worry out of proportion to a situation
Depression	Prolonged sadness or dejection
Homicidal ideation (HI)	Thoughts of killing others
Suicidal ideation (SI)	Thoughts of killing oneself
Insomnia	Difficulty falling or staying asleep

The 11 systems so far listed represent the core systems used in most ROS templates, and the remaining systems are covered next. A "complete" ROS for billing purposes includes 10 or more systems, which still applies to the ER (but not the clinic >2021).

12. Hematologic

Medical Term	Definition
Easy bleeding	More bleeding than expected with minor trauma
Easy bruising	Bruising appearing with minor or unknown trauma

13. Endocrine

The endocrine system refers to functions controlled by glands and hormones.

Medical Term	Definition
Intolerance to heat or cold	Feeling hot or cold out of proportion to the actual temperature, suggestive of thyroid dysfunction
Changes in hair or weight	Suggestive of thyroid dysfunction
Polyuria	Excessive urination

Polydipsia	Excessive thirst or liquid intake
Polyphagia	Excessive hunger or food intake

Polyuria, polydipsia, and polyphagia (the three P's) can be indicative of high blood sugar. Since high sugars may not be obvious to the patient at first, this is an example of how screening questions can aid in early diagnosis.

14. Allergic / Immunologic

This system refers to allergies and other abnormal responses of the immune system. Questions asked here may refer to environmental allergens (e.g., pollen, dust), food allergens (e.g., peanuts, eggs), and contact allergens (e.g., soap, hygiene products), or issues with frequent infections.

Medical Term	Definition
Rash	Redness or irritation of the skin
Pruritus	Itching or itchiness
Lymphadenopathy	Enlarged lymph nodes or "swollen nodes," common locations include the neck (cervical), armpits (axillary), and groin (inguinal)
Sneezing	Self-explanatory
Itchy or watery eyes	Self-explanatory

Because the HPI and ROS are intertwined, let's look at an example for abdominal pain. Note the italicized items and how they connect to the ROS.

History of Present Illness:
Jane Doe is a 38 y.o. female who presents with LLQ *abdominal pain*. She woke up with *malaise* yesterday morning and by evening developed localized left lower quadrant pain. She tried Pepto Bismol without relief and went to bed. Today the pain has been constant and gradually worsening throughout the day. She had a bowel movement 1 hour PTA with a small amount of *blood*.

Upon arrival, the pain is dull, non-radiating, rated 3-4/10, and nothing makes it better or worse. Denies *fever or chills*. Last BM before tonight was two days ago and *normal*. Her last menstrual period was a few days ago and unremarkable; current pain is different than her typical menstrual cramping. No *vaginal bleeding* or *discharge* since then. No history of hemorrhoids, ovarian cysts, or diverticulitis.

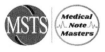

Review of Systems:
Constitutional: Denies fever or chills. + malaise.
Respiratory: Denies cough
Cardiovascular: Denies chest pain
Genitourinary: Denies vaginal bleeding or discharge
Gastrointestinal: + abdominal pain, hematochezia per HPI.

Semi-Subjective Sections

Medications, Allergies, and Past Medical and Surgical Histories may be purely subjective, reported by the patient, but may also draw on information objectively entered into the EHR. Mixed accuracy can occur, where the patient states they are taking X medication, but the EHR says Y. The patient may deny a history of surgeries, forgetting they had an appendectomy until the provider notices the scar on exam. Similarly, a provider may have entered "coronary artery disease" as a past diagnosis based on patient report, but later it is learned from medical records that the patient actually had a stroke.

The EHR has specific sections to enter these sections of history so that the information can be carried forward from visit to visit. They cannot be entered free-text, but instead are matched to lists of discrete data entries that enable better data capture and reporting. There might be a drop-down list to choose from, or a field where you begin typing the first few letters, and the software gives you a list of closely matching entries from which to choose. The EHR data entries can then be pulled into the note semi-automatically, by putting in special codes or characters into the medical record. This saves time typing the same past medical history at every visit but has a couple of downsides: 1) the note is bloated with too much clutter or irrelevant information, and 2) inaccurate information might be perpetuated indefinitely. Nevertheless, a great scribe reviews these sections and notices any discrepancies between the pre-filled EHR entries and what transpires between the provider and patient at that visit.

EHRs may have a button or check-mark to explicitly indicate that these sections have been reviewed by the provider, which should be checked if available. Some providers prefer to simply document that they have reviewed the information rather than pull it all into the note, to avoid clutter.

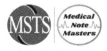

Medications

The provider's medical assistant or nurse typically reviews and updates the patient's medication list during the rooming process, but the physician may review the full medication list or just the highlights with the patient during the visit. This list should include both prescriptions and over-the-counter medications, and is often called the "home" medication list or outpatient med list. Patients are often confused about what medications they are taking or are supposed to be taking, so carefully reviewing the med list is essential in preventing medication errors. The process of

reviewing medications pre-visit and after-visit is called Medication Reconciliation, ("med rec") and is often a component of healthcare quality measures. After med rec is completed, the patient can receive a printout at discharge with the status of all of the recent medications, such as discontinuing one blood pressure medication and starting another.

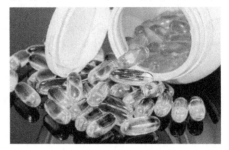

The EHR tracks medication orders from within the same healthcare system and can often import the medication history from other sources, so it is seldom necessary to type out all of the medication details manually. Typically, there are also pick-lists or smart fields in the EHR that populate lists of medications with common dosages to avoid typing out data free-text, where typos may occur.

1. Medication name – medications typically have a generic and brand name. Generic medication names are written in all lower-case letters (e.g., warfarin), and brand names are written with the first letter capitalized (e.g., Coumadin). Brand names are often easier to pronounce, so the patient may use the brand name, but the generic is listed or vice versa.

2. Route – the method by which the medication is delivered to the body. Medications may be administered orally (PO), intramuscularly (IM), intravenously (IV), or sublingually (beneath the tongue; SL). Nearly all medications taken at home are in the oral form, and therefore this may not be specified.

3. Dose – the amount of medication taken at any one time. Most medicines are dosed in milligrams (mg), but some may be micrograms or others.

4. Frequency – the number of times per day that a patient takes the medication. Abbreviations QD, BID, TID, and QID are used instead of the words once daily, twice daily, three times daily, and four times daily. The combination of dose and frequency is called "dosage."

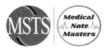

5. Quantity – the number of pills or amount of liquid prescribed in total for that prescription. Commonly, #30, #90, or 250mL.
6. Refills – the number of times the prescription can be reobtained from the pharmacy before requiring a new prescription.
7. Compliance – if a patient has a medication prescribed, it does not necessarily mean that the patient takes it as instructed. This is termed "non-compliant," and there may be a section in the EHR to denote compliance.
8. Active vs. Historical – most EHRs allow viewing of both active/current meds and meds that the patient took in the past then stopped. Antibiotics are a common example of a "historical" medication since they are taken short-term. Other historical meds might be pertinent to review, so the provider can identify what medications have already been attempted.

Medications:

Medication	Dosage	Quantity	Refills
Amoxicillin (historical, 6/2/18)	500 mg po TID	21	0
aspirin (OTC)	81 mg QD	-	-
omeprazole (Prilosec)	20 mg QD	30	2
simvastatin (Zocor)	20 mg QD	90	2

Allergies

Medication allergies are essential documentation, and most EHRs recognize this as a required field. Food allergies such as peanuts and eggs can be medically pertinent as well, and should be entered in the same section.

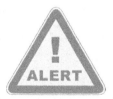

A medication allergy is different than a side effect. Allergic reactions involve hypersensitivity reactions from the immune system. They often include symptoms such as hives, rash, swelling, trouble breathing, and can progress to severe complications quickly. Medication side effects usually involve other symptoms like stomach upset or fatigue, for instance. Sometimes this section of the medical note contains side effects the patient reports as an allergy or vice versa, so the provider may have to ask clarifying questions. These should be carefully documented since any mistakes in this area could lead to serious problems.

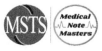

Past Medical History (PMHx)

The past medical history includes all medical diagnoses for the patient, and can include chronic medical problems currently present. Like other histories, the information can be entered free-text into the note, but more often the EHR has a specific section to enter discrete diagnoses that map to a code, which can then be copied into the note. For complex patients, this list may include dozens of different conditions entered by various healthcare roles over time, often becoming cluttered with duplication and accumulated outdated entries. The terms "Problem list" or "Health Concerns" are related terms used to include medical and non-medical issues like homelessness. For training purposes, we combine these concepts.

When appropriate, each listing will specify if the issue is acute or chronic. Listing a brief comment in the past medical history next to a particular condition can be very helpful for future healthcare professionals when they review a patient's chart. An example of a patient's past medical history and problem list may appear like this:

Past Medical History:

Diagnosis	Date	Comments
Hypertension		
Breast lump	2011	s/p lumpectomy, no recurrence
Hodgkin's disease	2011	Dx 2011 via biopsy, tx chemo and radiation; in remission
Tobacco use disorder		
LVH (left ventricular hypertrophy)	2013	echo 9/3/2015 with moderate LVH, EF 50%
CAD (coronary artery disease)	6/12/2013	80% stenosis of distal right coronary artery, tx'd with drug-eluting stent
Distal radius fracture, left	2009	

Problem List:

Problem	Comments
Hypertension	On amlodipine, metoprolol
Tobacco use disorder	1 ppd smoker
CAD (coronary artery disease)	s/p distal RCA stenting; annual FU with cardiology

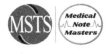

Past Surgical History (PSHx)

The past surgical history is sometimes regarded as a part of the past medical history, or it may be a separate section of the note altogether. It is an accounting of all surgeries and procedures the patient has had in the past. The term "status post," abbreviated "s/p" is often used to indicate the patient has undergone a procedure.

Surgical History:

Coronary stent 2013
Open reduction internal fixation (ORIF), left radius 2009
s/p appendectomy age 19

Some primary care providers focus on women's health, and may add a separate section for obstetric or gynecologic histories. Below is an example of gynecologic history entry in an EHR on the left, or free text on the right.

Gynecological History					**Gyn History**
Date of LMP		📅		📄 NOTE	LMP: hyst 2014
Date of last Pap smear		📅		📄 NOTE	Birth control: hyst
If post menopausal, age at menopause				📄 NOTE	Sexually active: no
HPV vaccine	Yes	No		📄 NOTE	Last pap: 2014, wnl
Sexually active	Yes	No		📄 NOTE	Abnormal pap: 1997, s/p LEEP
Sexual problems	Yes	No		📄 NOTE	STI: + condyloma, inactive
STIs/STDs	Yes	No		📄 NOTE	Mammogram: 7/1/20, wnl
					Colonoscopy: 8/1/19
					Bone density: never

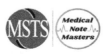

Healthcare Maintenance

Primary care providers are tasked with keeping an up-to-date record of a patient's screening exams (e.g., mammograms). In some cases, it is included in the past medical history such as the gynecologic history above, and other EHRs have a dedicated section of the note titled "Healthcare Maintenance" or "Preventative Care" or "Screening." This section serves as a running list of screening tests and may appear in an EHR as in the figure, or in free text as below:

Colonoscopy – last 2012 w/ 1 x tubular adenoma, repeat q5y
Mammogram – normal in 2016, 2020
Pap smear – with HPV co-testing, negative in 2017, repeat q5y

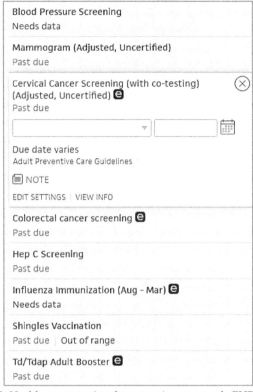

Figure 3.2: Healthcare screening data entry in an example EHR

Social History (SHx)

A patient's social history can be a highly variable section of the note. It may describe medically relevant habits (smoking, alcohol, and drug use), as well as associated information like the patient's living or financial situation. Some of these items are not always medically essential but are pertinent to care and establishing a good doctor-patient relationship. For example, if an elderly patient has had a recent fall, it is pertinent to know if the patient lives alone at home or in an assisted living facility. A patient's occupation may influence activity restrictions or safety issues, and occupation or hobbies like athletics come into play regarding injuries or rehab.

Like other historical elements, some components may be documented free-text in the HPI when pertinent to the HPI, but also documented in the specific EHR section dedicated to social history. Some examples of social history include:

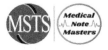

- Alcohol and other drug use (none, social drinker, h/o cocaine abuse, etc.)
- Marital or relationship status
- Living situation
- Occupation or physical requirements of work
- Athletic or other hobbies, dietary preferences

Smoking status is often addressed more specifically because it is tracked as a measure of quality care in many healthcare venues. The EHR typically has a designated section to document how much and how often the patient smokes, for how long, and what recommendations or assistance has been provided to help quit. "Pack-years" are most commonly used to describe smoking history, so a person who smokes 1 pack/day for 20 years has a "20 pack/year" history.

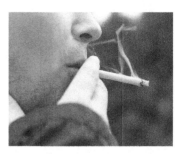

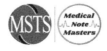

Figure 3.3: Smoking documentation in one EHR

Family History (FHx, FamHx)

The family history may or may not be pertinent to the patient's Reason for Visit and can be simply omitted or recorded as "non-contributory." However, for other visits like a screening physical, it may reveal risk factors that need to be addressed. The medical history of first-degree relatives (parent, sibling, or child) is most pertinent, but the provider may also expand out to second-degree relatives (aunt, uncle, grandmother, grandfather). In the ER, family history is most often addressed in light of risk for cardiovascular diseases like heart disease, stroke, or blood clotting disorders that impact morbidity risk for the ER RFV. For instance, a history of coronary artery disease in the patient's father at age 52, pulmonary embolism in the patient's mother, or a sister with severe lupus.

The most common conditions addressed in the family medical history are listed below, because they often run in families and have genetic risk factors. Colon, breast, and prostate cancers are especially significant in the primary clinic, as they will affect the age or frequency at which a patient needs screening.

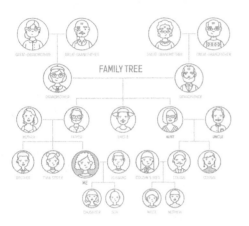

- Diabetes mellitus
- Hypertension
- Hyperlipidemia
- Heart attack – this is most important for first-degree male family members before age 55 and first-degree female family members before age 65.
- Stroke
- Colon cancer
- Breast cancer
- Prostate cancer (males only)

Now that we have collected all of the information needed from the subjective section, the provider will move on to the physical exam. This may be the point in the visit where the provider gets up from a chair to perform the exam, which is your clue to change gears. However, most providers will continue to ask historical questions concurrently with the exam to keep conversation going, so your note-taking will need to bounce back and forth between the Subjective and Objective sections.

End of Chapter Quiz

1. Which answer below would be an unacceptable chief complaint?
   a. Urinary tract infection
   b. Dysuria
   c. Urinary frequency
   d. Cough
   e. Follow-up hypertension
2. Which is a more technical term for "fainting?"
   a. Emesis
   b. Dyspnea
   c. Malaise
   d. Syncope
3. Which answer is NOT a description of the quality of pain?
   a. Sharp
   b. Severe
   c. Burning
   d. Dull
4. Which symptom is NOT part of the constitutional system in the ROS?
   a. Malaise
   b. Fever
   c. Fatigue
   d. All of the above are part of the constitutional system
5. Most patients can relay all medications and dosage accurately.
   a. True
   b. False
6. Chief Complaint and Reason for Visit are the same.
   a. True
   b. False
7. A medication side effect is the same as an allergy.
   a. True
   b. False

Answers: 1. A 2. D 3. B 4. D 5. B 6. A 7. B

4. The Physical Exam

The next major task for the medical scribe is accurate documentation of the provider's physical exam. The physical exam portion of the note represents the provider's findings based primarily on what they see, feel, and hear. Because it is written from the perspective of the provider, it is written almost entirely in medical terms. So, while a patient may report the symptom of shortness of breath, the provider would observe a patient struggling to breathe and say, "The patient is in moderate respiratory distress" or "Patient exhibits increased work of breathing." Symptoms do not generally belong in the physical exam unless it is a symptom the provider has elicited by a physical exam maneuver. The interpretation of any abnormal findings is discussed in the MDM section of the note (covered later), not in the exam itself. Hence, there are no diagnoses in the exam section either.

Some providers will choose to narrate findings to their scribe as they perform the exam, and others will summarize abnormal findings after leaving the patient's room. This is usually a matter of preference, though sometimes it can be insensitive to discuss certain findings within the patient's presence. Just like the HPI, make sure to note any limitations to the exam, such as if a provider indicates that the abdominal exam was limited by obesity, or if the TM was obscured by cerumen.

Your goal as a scribe is to observe the provider's examinations and then document the appropriate finding(s) accurately and thoroughly. For example, when physicians use an otoscope to look into a patient's ear, what are they looking at? What should you write in the note? In this section, we will outline and describe each part of the routine physical exam, along with some of the most common findings.

The physical exam can be divided into activities based on a provider's senses:
1. Inspection – visual observation
2. Palpation – maneuvering, feeling, pressing or pushing on the body part being examined
3. Auscultation – listening, typically with a stethoscope
4. Percussion – tapping on the body part being examined and potentially listening for the quality of sound produced (less commonly performed)
5. The sense of smell is not commonly applied, but is sometimes used to describe the smell of a wound or a patient's breath.

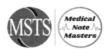

Taste is no longer applicable, but in the Middle Ages, physicians tasted urine for a sweet taste, associated with diabetes mellitus (mellitus = sweet).

As a rule of thumb, you can assume that a particular examination lacks abnormal findings unless the provider indicates otherwise. However, it is not accurate or specific to write the word "normal" for an exam section, since this does not specify what exactly was examined or what portions of the exam were normal. For **individual** exam elements, terms such as "within normal limits," "clear," or "unremarkable" can be used, but would not be appropriate for the whole section. Therefore, when you see the provider look in the patient's ears with the otoscope, you would write:

ENT: TMs clear bilaterally. External canals unremarkable.
not
ENT: normal

Eventually, you should be able to do this for all of the most commonly examined sections, including:

- General appearance
- Ear, Nose, Throat (ENT) or Head, Eyes, Ears, Nose and Throat (HEENT)
- Neck
- Respiratory
- Cardiovascular
- Abdomen
- Neurological
- Extremities
- Skin
- Area of the chief complaint

The physical exam is documented in a head-to-toe manner, regardless of the position of the patient.

The exam may be comprehensive (including genital and rectal exams during an annual physical), or it may be comprised of only a couple of focused exam sections, depending on the chief complaint.

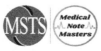

4. The Physical Exam

The following example demonstrates a normal physical exam including some commonly used abbreviations, so you are familiar with them. Most providers/scribes have a "normal" exam template built into the EHR that includes the exam pieces that provider performs on a routine basis, and no abbreviations are necessary. Remember that templates and other "prefills" can lead to problems, usually including exam pieces that were not done or omitting abnormal findings. Depending on the EHR, the vital signs entered during the intake process can be pulled into the note fairly easily.

Vital Signs: Heart Rate: 80, Respiratory Rate: 14, Blood Pressure: 120/80, Oximetry: 99% on room air, Temperature: 98.6°F

General:	Patient appears well, resting comfortably, no acute distress (NAD)
HEENT:	Normocephalic, atraumatic (NC, AT). Pupils equal, round, reactive to light (PERRL), extraocular movements intact (EOMI). Conjunctiva well-perfused, nonicteric. Moist mucus membranes. Oropharynx without erythema or swelling. Tonsillar pillars within normal limits (WNL). Uvula is midline. Good dentition. Tympanic membranes (TMs) clear bilaterally.
Neck:	Supple with full range of motion (ROM). No cervical lymphadenopathy (LAD). No thyromegaly or nodules.
Cardiovascular:	Regular rate and rhythm (RRR). No gallops, rubs or murmurs (m/g/r). Pulses intact x four extremities. Good capillary refill.
Respiratory:	Clear to auscultation (CTA) bilaterally, good air movement.
Abdomen:	Soft, non-tender, non-distended (NT, ND) without organomegaly. Normoactive bowel sounds (NABS).
Neurological:	Alert and oriented (A&O), facial and extremity movements symmetric, ambulatory.
Psychiatric:	Normal speech, normal affect.
Skin:	Exposed skin is unremarkable. No rashes.
Musculoskeletal:	No lower extremity edema. No midline or lumbar paraspinal tenderness.

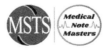

Note that for each category, at least a couple items are specified. In the Billing & Coding chapter, you will learn that the number of categories and the number of elements listed affect reimbursement based on 1995-2020 guidelines for clinics and current guidelines for the ER, and most exam templates are built on this premise. Also note that the phrases used are a combination of POSITIVE findings, stating what is seen or heard, and NEGATIVES that denote findings that are lacking. These positives and negatives together shape the clinical decision making as to what is likely or unlikely to be going on with the patient.

A common mistake for both providers and scribes is to confuse right vs. left, since the provider is facing the patient, and the scribe may be in another position. The laterality of any exam finding should be very clearly indicated in the documentation – mixups can lead to embarrassment and potentially horrible consequences.

Some EHRs have the capability to document in a more visual fashion. A schematic drawing of the face might be pictured for instance, and the location of a lesion can be drawn onto the figure rather than attempting to describe the precise location and size with words. Some EHRs are formatted with click-boxes rather than free text, as depicted in the figure. Resist the temptation to click a generic "normal" vs "abnormal," which may be too nonspecific to be informative. Remember documentation makes no assumptions, and if it isn't documented, it didn't happen, so be specific about what exactly was examined and what was found or not.

Physical Examination M <Hide Structure> <Use Dictate> <Use Free Text>

VS/Measurements >>	Vital signs from flowsheet		
	3/23/2011 4:27 PM CDT	Temperature Oral	37.0 DegC
		Peripheral Pulse Rate	78 bpm
		Respiratory Rate	14 br/min
		Systolic Blood Pressure	131 mmHg
		Diastolic Blood Pressure	77 mmHg
		Mean Arterial Pressure, Cuff	95 mmHg
	Measurements from flowsheet		
	3/23/2011 4:27 PM CDT	Height/Length Measured	185.00 cm
		Weight Measured	78.000 kg
	/ Document vital signs+ / OTHER		
General>>	Alert and oriented / No acute distress / Mild distress / Moderate distress / Severe distress / OTHER		
HENT >>	NAD / Normocephalic / No sinus tenderness / Normal hearing / Moist oral mucosa / OTHER		
Respiratory>>	NAD / Lungs CTA / Non-labored respirations / BS equal / Symmetrical expansion / No chest wall tenderness / OTHER		
Cardiovascular>>	Normal rate / Regular rhythm / No murmur / No gallop / Good pulses equal in all extremities / Normal peripheral perfusion / No edema / OTHER		
Gastrointestinal M >>	Soft / Non-tender / Non-distended / Normal bowel sounds / No organomegaly / OTHER		
Lymphatics >>	No lymphadenopathy neck, axilla, groin / OTHER		

Figure 4.1: Example of click-based exam entry in an EHR

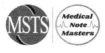

In this chapter, we will break down the exam piece-by-piece with explanations of common terminology. Because physical exam maneuvers are difficult to describe in text, the associated online course videos are recommended alongside this chapter to reinforce learning.

The Vital Signs (VS)

Vital signs are quantitative measures of a patient's core bodily processes (hence the term vital), mainly reflecting cardiovascular (heart and blood vessels) and pulmonary (lung) function. The five vital signs include the patient's blood pressure (BP), heart rate (HR), respiratory rate (RR), oxygen saturation (oximetry), and temperature (T). Not all patients will need to have all vital signs documented (such as blood pressure on a toddler). Vital signs will usually be entered into the EHR during the rooming process and may be easy to overlook. However, remember that prefilled EHR information needs to be reviewed for accuracy. It is not uncommon for someone to enter a typo that will be pulled into your note without paying close attention. Further, any abnormality in VS should be rechecked during the visit, the new results documented, and reasoning discussed in clinical decision-making.

Heart Rate (HR)

Heart rate is the number of beats per minute (bpm) of the heart, which tends to be higher for infants and children. For adults, greater than 100 bpm is generally considered abnormally high (tachycardia) during a doctor's visit, since presumably, the patient is not exercising. In contrast, bradycardia is a slow heart rate, around 50-60 bpm, but this is normal in some people and asymptomatic in many. HR is most commonly measured alongside oximetry with a finger probe as pictured, and/or may be assessed during the cardiovascular exam.

Oximetry (SpO2, SaO2)

Also known as pulse oximetry or "pulse ox," SpO2 or SaO2, this measures the oxygenation of the blood. Using a small probe attached to the patient's finger (or elsewhere), pulse oximetry estimates the percentage of oxygenated hemoglobin based on measured light 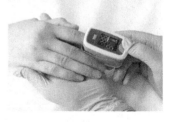 wavelengths. Less than 90% is low and called **hypoxia**. Next to the measurement should be an indication of what air the patient was breathing at the time of the analysis: room air (RA), supplemental oxygen like 2L of O2 per nasal cannula (NC), or higher amounts of O2.

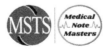

Blood Pressure (BP)

These numbers represent the arterial blood pressure during systole (systolic blood pressure, SBP) and diastole, respectively. It is usually verbalized as two numbers, so a BP of 140/90 is stated as "140 over 90." It is most commonly measured with automated cuffs, though it can be measured manually. When the BP is consistently 140/90 in a calm

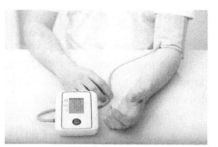

situation, it is considered abnormally high. However, some factors can lead to slightly elevated readings, such as tensing the arm, using too small a cuff, or just being stressed at the physician's office, called "white coat" hypertension. When the SBP falls below 90, it could be abnormally low, called hypotension, or could be relatively normal for that patient. Like most numbers in medicine, the number is more valuable when interpreted in context.

Respiratory Rate (RR)

Respiratory rate is the number of breaths per minute. Less than 12 is a slow rate and is called bradypnea, and greater than 20 breaths per minute is fast, called **tachypnea** (reasonably common). RR is rarely taken through automated devices and the value may be estimated simply by watching the patient's breathing.

Temperature (T)

Most temperature measurements are close estimates of the core body temperature. Temperature can be measured orally, rectally, in the axilla, or by using an ear or forehead device with touchless infrared technology. The method by which a temperature reading is obtained is usually stated next to the number itself. Science uses the metric system, so the temperature is often reported in Celsius with the Fahrenheit conversion alongside for ease of familiarity. Average body temperature is approximately or 37°C or 98.6°F, but can normally range a degree or so on either side. To be considered a fever, the temperature must be higher than 38°C (100.4°F).

Height/Weight

Height and weight are commonly listed in the same section as the vital signs. Due to the obesity epidemic, weight management has emerged as a quality measure for primary care, including monitoring BMI (body mass index, BMI = kg/m^2) as a risk factor for multiple conditions.

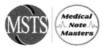

Adult Physical Exam

General Appearance

The physical exam begins with a general section designed to capture the first impressions of the patient. This part of the exam is documented in almost every patient and includes some common descriptors listed below. Remember to document items that might seem obvious at the time.

- Appearance – well-groomed, disheveled, angry, cooperative, sweating, fearful, smells of EtOH
- Body habitus – well-developed, well-nourished, thin, obese
- Comfort level – comfortable, uncomfortable
- Body position – seated, lying down, pacing, rocking back/forth
- Level of distress – most physical exam templates include the phrase "no acute distress (NAD)" to denote that the patient does not appear to need immediate medical attention.

Head, Eyes, Ears, Nose, and Throat (HEENT) Exam

This section of the physical exam is a combination of several anatomically adjacent regions. It is primarily examined in its entirety for patients who have a chief complaint that involves the head, eyes, ears, nose, or throat (like a sore throat). Sometimes the eyes and head may be listed separately in the physical exam, and the remaining sections will form the ENT (ears, nose, and throat) exam.

Head ("H" of HEENT)

- Normocephalic (NC) –a normally-shaped and sized head
- Atraumatic (AT) – no signs of head trauma (like bruising or a laceration)
- Pupils are equal, round, and reactive to light (abbreviated PERRL) – the pupils constrict (shrink) symmetrically and appropriately in response to light, such as a small penlight
- Sclera anicteric – no icterus, or yellowing, of the sclera (white of the eye)
- Extraocular muscles are intact (EOMI) without nystagmus – the muscles controlling eye (ocular) movement are functioning well. If specifically examined (rather than just watching the patient's eye movement during conversation), the provider will have the patient follow a pattern of movement in front of the patient's eyes. If the eye muscles are miscoordinated, the patient may experience double vision or dizziness, which is a rare instance when symptoms are allowed in the PE. In movies,

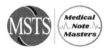

this exam maneuver is often depicted during sobriety tests, since nystagmus, or quivering eye movement, is seen while intoxicated.
- No conjunctival injection – injection refers to the presence of streaky redness
- Conjunctiva well-perfused – inspecting the inside of the lower lid to check color/perfusion

Ears ("E" of HEENT)

In the ear exam, the most important structure is the tympanic membrane (TM), the translucent membrane that transmits sound to the middle and inner ear. The most common abnormality of a tympanic membrane comes from middle ear fluid or infection, which causes an ordinarily clear TM to appear red, dull, or bulging.

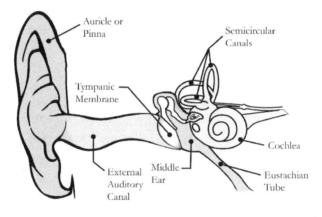

Figure 4.2: Ear anatomy

- TMs clear, light reflex intact – the TMs are normally nearly translucent or pearly with a reflective surface, but may become dull, erythematous, or even perforated from infections or trauma
- Middle ear effusion – the accumulation of fluid in the Eustachian tube behind the TM, which may be further described as clear, cloudy

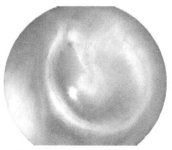

Figure 4.3: Normal TM appearance

The auditory canals may also be mentioned in the exam, and findings may include:
- External auditory canal is obstructed with cerumen (ear wax).
- External auditory canal is erythematous with purulent discharge—red with discharge, as might be seen in swimmer's ear.

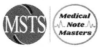

Nose ("N" of HEENT)

Examination of the nose is typically only performed in patients with a related chief complaint. Within each nostril are three bony structures called turbinates that affect air movement, and a septum dividing the right and left sides. The mucus membranes of the turbinates may bleed causing epistaxis, or with inflammation/infection become erythematous, edematous, or produce rhinorrhea.

Throat ("T" of HEENT)

The throat exam includes the examination of the oral cavity (i.e., the mouth) and the oropharynx (the throat), which typically occurs when a physician asks a patient to open up and say "ah." For sore throat complaints, the uvula and tonsils will be noted. Tonsillar size is graded from 0 (small, not swollen) to 4+ (very large and obstructive). Strep throat (i.e. strep pharyngitis) is a common condition that may present with swollen tonsils (e.g., 2+ tonsils), tonsillar exudate (pus), and erythema of the posterior oropharynx.

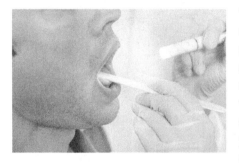

The patient's hydration status may be addressed by writing "moist mucus membranes" (MMM) to indicate an average saliva moisture amount. This denotes that the patient seems adequately hydrated, whereas dry mucus membranes might suggest the patient is dehydrated. The provider may also note that the uvula is midline, no lesions are seen, that the soft palate elevates appropriately, or that the gingiva are well-perfused. Any voice changes may be noted here or in the General section, such as hoarseness, or denoted as "phonation strong" when the voice is normal volume and pitch.

Dental exam

The dental exam is also included in the HEENT section of the physical exam and is performed during the evaluation of the oral cavity. For patients without a dental complaint, the exam may state "dentition in good repair" or similar, as opposed to diffusely poor dentition seen in some medical conditions. Each tooth is assigned a particular number by the tooth numbering system shown, which is important for patients with dental complaints.

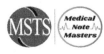

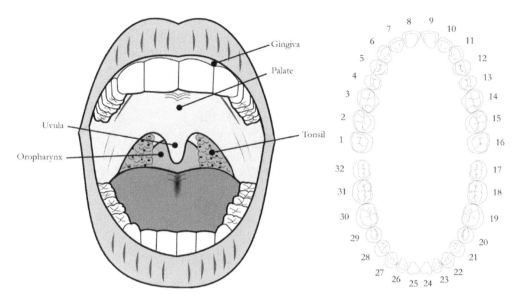

Figure 4.4: Throat and oral cavity; dental numbering

Neck Exam

The neck exam usually involves inspection, range of motion testing, palpation of the cervical lymph nodes, and palpation of the paraspinous/paraspinal muscles for those with neck pain. Less commonly, the physician will assess cardiovascular issues by examining for jugular vein distention (JVD) or narrowing of the carotid artery. A narrowed artery can produce an abnormal sound called a bruit due to turbulent flow and is one of the few times a physician will auscultate directly over the neck. If you see the physician specially position the patient and look closely or measure veins on the side of the neck, this is likely an exam for JVD. Like many sections of the physical exam, the neck exam is not performed on all patients.

- Supple – no stiffness or restriction in range of motion.
- Tenderness – pain upon palpation. It is relatively common to have tenderness over the muscles on either side of the neck (paraspinous or paraspinal muscles) as well as the trapezius muscles.
- No thyromegaly – enlargement of the thyroid gland in the anterior lower neck. You will know the physician is performing this exam if the patient is asked to swallow while the physician palpates this area.
- No lymphadenopathy (LAD), or just adenopathy– refers to abnormalities (or lack thereof) of lymph nodes. Palpation for lymph nodes is commonly

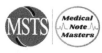

assessed in conjunction with infectious complaints since lymph nodes react and swell to infections in their vicinity. The primary lymph nodes in the neck region include the submandibular nodes, anterior cervical lymph nodes, and posterior cervical lymph nodes.

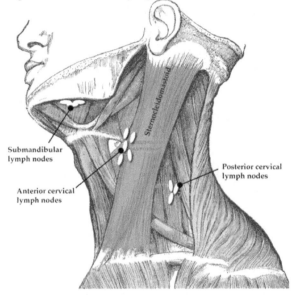

Figure 4.5: Cervical lymph nodes

Chest or Respiratory Exam

The respiratory exam, sometimes referred to as the chest or thorax exam, is primarily focused on the auscultation of the lungs. To examine the patient's lungs, the provider will ask the patient to take deep breaths in and out as they move the stethoscope over regions on the chest and upper back. The unremarkable exam may include these descriptors:

- Clear to auscultation bilaterally– no abnormal breath sounds
- Good air movement – in contrast to diminished or reduced breath sounds
- Speaking full sentences – indicates the patient has normal work of breathing

Many abnormalities heard during auscultation occur because of the narrowing of the air passages (also known as the bronchial tree), which makes typically smooth or streamlined airflow become turbulent. Each of the four major lung sounds listed below corresponds to the narrowing of a particular part of the bronchial tree and can, therefore, be diagnostically helpful in discerning the underlying cause of a

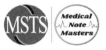

patient's symptoms. Like most physical exam abnormalities, the note should specify the location and timing, which in this case would be the region of the lung and inspiratory or expiratory timing. Since any respiratory abnormality could be an indicator of a risky underlying process, additional descriptors are helpful to give the reader a sense of how concerning the patient's respiratory status is. For instance, a patient with underlying lung disease may have decreased breath sounds at baseline and may seem well, conversant and relaxed, so the concern level is lower than for a patient with new findings struggling to finish sentences.

- Wheezes – high-pitched, whistling
- Crackles (or rales) – tiny popping sounds, can be fine or coarse, Velcro-like
- Rhonchi – low-pitched, coarse
- Stridor – a high-pitched sound from the upper airway, often seen in croup
- Diminished air movement – poor air movement in and out of the lungs with breathing, which makes it difficult to hear abnormal lung sounds on exam.
- If a cough is heard, it may be described as dry, barky, wheezy, loose, rattly, or other descriptors

Cardiovascular Exam

The cardiovascular exam includes examination of the patient's heart and vascular system. It consists of auscultation over the patient's anterior chest wall (i.e., heart) in several locations (e.g., the left and right sternal borders) and may also include an examination of peripheral circulation if pertinent. As a scribe, it can be difficult to discern if a provider is auscultating a patient's heart or lungs because both involve placement of the stethoscope on the chest. The major difference is that a full lung exam is auscultated from the posterior thorax. Providers also ask the patient to take deep breaths through the mouth during the lung exam, and they ask the patient to breathe normally or softly to auscultate the heart. Typically, the provider is listening to both heart and lungs during chest auscultation so document both exam sections.

Auscultation Terms

- Regular rate and rhythm (RRR) –a regular rate describes normal speed and timing of the heartbeat, and the rhythm refers to the pattern of the beats.
- No murmurs, gallops, or rubs – no abnormal or extra heart sounds. If the patient does have a murmur, then the location and timing should be documented. The provider will specify right upper sternal border, left upper sternal border, left lower sternal border, or the apex. It will also be noted whether it is heard during systole or diastole, as well as the severity.

Pulses

In a focused physical exam, the physician will typically only check the pulses distal to an injury (e.g., the radial pulse in a patient with a forearm laceration). In patients with CHF or peripheral vascular disease (PVD), the physician may check several pulses as listed below. PVD patients often have decreased pulses at baseline, so previous notes may need review.

- Dorsalis pedis (or pedal)
- Posterior tibial (PT)
- Femoral
- Radial
- Brachial
- Carotid

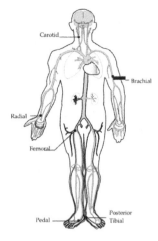

Figure 4.6: Peripheral pulses

Pulse strength may be documented as "strong" or "normal and symmetric" or graded from 0 to 4+.

- 0   absent (not palpable)
- 1+   diminished
- 2+   normal
- 3+   increased
- 4+   bounding

Capillary refill

Like palpation of the distal pulses, assessing capillary refill times is a metric of a patient's blood flow to the distal extremities (fingers and toes, mainly). The physician may squeeze the patient's fingernail, temporarily shutting off blood supply to the nail and turning it white; this is called blanching. The physician will then release pressure and watch as blood returns to the blanched area, and if it takes less than 2 seconds, it is considered normal.

Abdominal (GI) Exam

The abdominal or gastrointestinal (GI) exam is primarily examined via palpation and auscultation, but may also be assessed via inspection for distention, scars, or signs of trauma, and via percussion for abnormal air or fluid. Because each quadrant overlies particular abdominal organs, tenderness localized to a single quadrant can

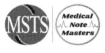

be very helpful in discerning the cause of a patient's symptoms. Overall, the unremarkable abdominal exam may include these components:

- Soft – in contrast to a hard or firm abdomen
- Non-distended – abdomen is not tense or bulging
- Non-tender – palpation does not cause discomfort
- No rebound– more fully known as rebound tenderness, is examined by steadily applying pressure to an area, then suddenly releasing the pressure
- No guarding – guarding is the voluntary or involuntary flexion of the abdominal muscles by the patient during palpation to minimize exam discomfort

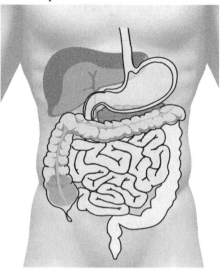

- Normoactive bowel sounds (NABS) – examined via auscultation, in contrast to absent bowel sounds or hyperactive bowel sounds
- No organomegaly, or no hepatosplenomegaly (HSM) – enlarged organs are not palpated. Special maneuvers are required to palpate the liver or spleen under the edge of the rib cage, and the exam is often limited by obesity.
- No direct or indirect inguinal hernia palpable with cough

Rectal Exam

The rectal exam consists of external inspection to look for hemorrhoids, fissures, or other lesions and is followed by insertion of a single finger into the rectal vault called the digital rectal exam. The finger can palpate internal hemorrhoids as well as the size and uniformity of the prostate gland in males. Fecal residue obtained from the rectal exam can be tested for the presence of (occult) blood, which is valuable information in certain disorders. Common descriptions of the rectal exam include:

- No evidence for fistula or fissure, no external hemorrhoids.
- Normal appearing stool in rectal vault.
- Smooth, symmetric, non-tender prostate.

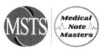

Genitourinary Exam

Male-organ Specific

The examination of the penis, scrotum, and testicles constitutes the male-organ genitourinary exam. The scribe may be excused from the room or asked to stand off to the side for the patient's privacy, and the provider will relay the findings later. An inguinal hernia is in the same vicinity, and the provider may assess for this while the patient is fully undressed, although the findings would be included in the GI exam. Normal exam findings may include:

- Normal external genitalia inspection without lesions
- No scrotal swelling. Testes smooth, symmetric and nontender.
- No blood or discharge at the urethral meatus
- Cremasteric reflex intact bilaterally

Pelvic Exam

The genitourinary examination in females is also called the pelvic exam. Because this is a personally sensitive exam, the scribe may be asked to step to the side for privacy. Most clinics do not allow GU exams to be performed 1:1 doctor: patient; instead, enforcing a "chaperone" policy whereby another person is always present to witness the encounter and ensure no impropriety occurs. If a chaperone is utilized, it should be documented.

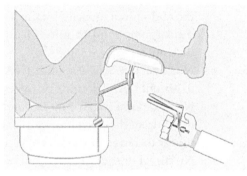

Figure 4.7: Positioning for a full pelvic exam, sometimes called "lithotomy"

The patient is asked to undress from the waist down, and then placed into position as pictured above to facilitate the exam. As with most exams, the pelvic exam begins with inspection. After visualizing the external genitalia, a speculum is inserted into the vagina and opened slightly to allow visualization of the vagina and cervix. Often a swab is used at this point to collect a sample from the cervix to be analyzed for infections and/or cancerous cells. Then palpation is performed with a bimanual exam, where the provider inserts two fingers into the vagina and uses the other hand to palpate the suprapubic area, such that the pelvic organs are in-between the two hands. Palpating internal organs is often challenging, especially in obese patients,

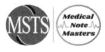

so any limitations should be documented. When an infection is a concern, the provider may manipulate the cervix to assess for cervical motion tenderness (CMT).

Normal pelvic exam findings may include:
- External genitalia without visible lesions
- Physiologic vaginal fluid within vault. Cervix nulliparous, wnl.
- No adnexal mass or tenderness. Negative CMT.

In pregnant patients, more descriptors of the cervix and uterus may be used, including uterine size and if dilation is palpable.
- Outer cervix soft, open to fingertip, inner os closed
- Uterus palpable 2cm above symphysis, fundus firm and nontender
- Cervix 1 cm dilated
- Scant dark maroon blood in vault, no active bleeding

Breast Exam

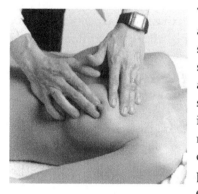

The clinical breast exam is an optional part of most annual physicals, where the breasts and surrounding tissues are inspected and palpated for signs of breast cancer. Inspection may reveal abnormalities such as breast size or shape changes, skin changes like dimpling or induration, or nipple irregularities that may be a sign of an underlying mass. Often, the patient is asked to lift her arm overhead, to spread the breast tissue for improved palpation. During palpation, the provider is evaluating for suspicious lumps or bumps in the breast tissue itself, as well as the neighboring lymph nodes in the axilla. Any abnormalities will be documented regarding size, mobility, location, depth, texture, and shape. Some breast exam findings may include:

- Breasts are symmetric, nontender, without palpable masses. No skin dimpling. No visual nipple irregularities or discharge. No axillary LAD.
- Bilateral breasts are firm with diffuse nodularity. No fixed or focal masses.
- R breast 2 o'clock linear 2cm surgical scar, unchanged from previous.

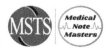

Neurological Exam

The "neuro" exam is typically performed in more comprehensive physical exams or in patients with neurological symptoms (e.g., slurred speech, altered mental status, etc.). The unremarkable neurological exam may include the terms below, but some special tests are omitted since they are infrequently performed.

- Alert – the patient responds to the environment and other stimuli
- Oriented times three – the patient can answer accurately to all three orientations (person, place, and time). When combined with "alert," it is written as A&O x3 and is the most basic test of cognitive function. You may also see it written as "the patient is oriented to person, place, month…" or another fact (like the season, president of the United States, etc.)
- Motor strength 5/5 (specify location) – Strength is graded from 0 to 5, with 0/5, meaning the patient has no muscle strength at all, while 5/5 is considered normally strong. Strength can be checked by providing resistance against the provider, such as pushing or pulling against the arms, or by certain movements such as being able to stand on tiptoes.
- Sensation intact (specify location) – sensation is checked by testing the patient's recognition of light touch or pinprick to various aspects of the face, arms and legs. In patients with diabetes, a specialized monofilament exam is used to test sensation in the feet as a means to screen for neuropathy.
- Cranial nerves II-XII grossly intact — the cranial nerves control function of several regions of the head and neck. Formal testing of each nerve is seldom done unless related to the patient's complaint, so a less specific phrase such as "facial movements symmetric" is more accurate.
- Deep Tendon Reflex (DTR) — reflexes are involuntary movements enacted at the level of the spinal cord, brought on by tapping the tendon. You likely immediately imagine a doctor tapping on a patient's knee with an involuntary kick to follow; however, this exam is not often performed. A normal exam may describe a reflex as intact and symmetric, or reflexes can also be recorded on a scale of 0-4 listed below.

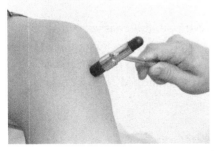

For example: "2/4 bilateral patellar reflexes" would represent normal patellar reflexes.
- ➢ 0 Absent
- ➢ 1+ Diminished
- ➢ 2+ Normal
- ➢ 3+ Increased, but no clonus
- ➢ 4+ Markedly hyperactive with clonus

Psychiatric Exam

The psychiatric exam is primarily based on a directed conversation with the patient, as well as observation of behavior. If the patient presents with a mental health complaint, then these observations should be recorded under the heading of the psychiatric exam. Some terms encountered may include:

- Hallucinations – seeing (visual) or hearing (auditory) things that are disconnected from reality
- Suicidal or homicidal ideation (SI or HI) – the intention of harming oneself or others. This is important to document for medicolegal reasons.
- Affect – depressed, sad, anxious, angry, labile, flattened
- Thoughts– logical, tangential, nonsensical, paranoid, perseverative
- Speech – clear, fast, slow, pressured, whispering, monotone
- Psychomotor – hyperactive, slowed

Skin, Integumentary or Dermatologic Exam

The skin exam for non-dermatologic complaints is often generically assessed as "Exposed skin is warm, dry, without rash or lesion," accomplished simply by looking at a patient's exposed skin without requiring specific examination. A dermatologic complaint would warrant further detail including the size, location, and pattern of the following findings:

- Abscess (subcutaneous) – a collection of pus beneath the epidermis
- Abrasion – superficial skin wound, a scrape
- Cyst – a sac-like collection of tissue or fluid
- Erythema or erythematous – redness
- Induration – firmness, thickening of the skin often from inflammation
- Fluctuance – term to describe a "squishy" feeling of a fluid collection
- Jaundice – yellowish discoloration of the skin
- Pale – skin lacks its usual color
- Macules – flat lesions
- Papules – raised lesions
- Maculopapular – a mixture of raised and flat regions
- Ulcers – skin breakdown
- Urticaria – hives
- Warmth – skin is warm to the touch, as opposed to hot or cold
- Bruising (contusion) – a collection of blood beneath the skin (hematoma) that dos not blanch, typically due to trauma

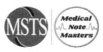

- o Petechiae – small (1-2 mm) spots
- o Purpura – medium (3-10 mm) red or purple spots
- o Ecchymosis – large (> 10 mm) hematomas; a typical bruise

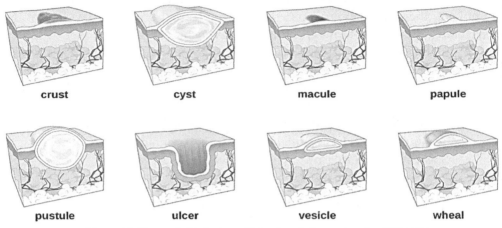

crust	cyst	macule	papule
pustule	ulcer	vesicle	wheal

Figure 4.8: Types of skin lesions. This photo is licensed under CC BY-SA

Musculoskeletal, Extremity, and/or Back Exam

The combination of terms or splitting them apart largely depends on what needs to be documented. For a medical patient, examining the lower extremities for edema might be most valuable, as opposed to a trauma patient that may need these categories split up even further. When multiple areas are examined, it is best to split up each location so that the exam findings do not run together and lead to indistinct documentation regarding site and laterality. Some findings may include:

- No cyanosis, clubbing, or edema (C/C/E) – a phrase for lack of cyanosis (blue discoloration of the skin), clubbing (a deformity of the fingernails), or edema
- Edema – accumulation of fluid within tissues, causing increased size. It may be called pitting edema and rated from 1+ (mild) to 4+ (severe).
- Crepitus – cracking or popping sounds
- Effusion – accumulation of fluid within a joint
- Range of motion (ROM) – a joint moving through its natural movements
- Spasm – involuntary contraction of a muscle
- Obvious deformities – visually deformed anatomic features

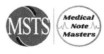

In the case of injuries, the circulation, motor, and sensory status of the region should be examined to detect possible vascular or neurologic injuries. The scribe may document these findings alongside the injury in the musculoskeletal section, or separately in the cardiovascular and neurologic sections. The specific element examined and the finding is documented, rather than nonspecific terms such as "intact" or "normal." If the initial exam is limited due to pain, it would be re-examined later. For a shoulder dislocation for instance, you would document the radial pulse, sensation around the upper arm/deltoid area, and muscular strength after relocation.

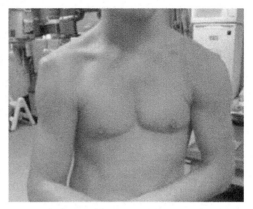

Figure 4.9: Obvious deformity due to a shoulder dislocation, which would also show decreased ROM and muscle spasm

The examination of the back may be included in the musculoskeletal exam or as a separate heading. The back exam includes examination of the thoracic, lumbar, and sacral regions of the back and spine. Strains of the large muscles that run alongside the spine grouped together as "paraspinous" or "paraspinal" muscles are the most common injury from lifting, twisting, shoveling or similar, and spasms may be palpable. Midline tenderness over the vertebral bodies is more concerning for a

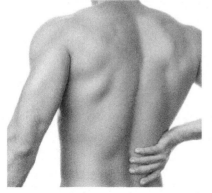

bony pathology, although spinal fractures are relatively uncommon outside of serious physical trauma or bone diseases. Like the shoulder example, the back exam often must be reassessed after pain medications when the patient is more comfortable, and associated neurologic findings are documented to verify the patient does not have a neurologic emergency called cauda equina (discussed later).

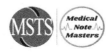

Pediatric Physical Exam

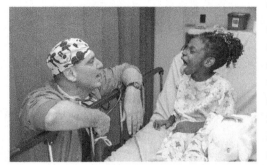

The pediatric physical exam is slightly different than the adult exam since children have several developmental differences from adults. Physically, there are many obvious differences, such as fontanelles ("soft spot") in infants. Emotionally, some children are unable to express symptoms or cooperate with the exam. Physiologically, children also tend to have different vital signs than adults and run fevers more often, so VS are carefully documented and interpreted on arrival and often rechecked. So, while the physician is using the same basic principles of assessment, he/she will be looking for different findings and the phraseology differs from the adult exam. You can also refer to the Well Child Check Section for more information about pediatric assessments.

General:

- The patient is non-toxic appearing – the child does not appear severely ill
- The child is playful, smiling, running around the exam room, etc. – a child's activity level helps demonstrate that the child is not seriously ill
- The child is crying but consolable by mother – often young children will cry while being examined but will stop when held by a parent
- Child interacting well with parents
- The child appears lethargic – this is a serious statement that the child has a significantly reduced energy level or level of consciousness

HEENT:

- Fontanels are flat – the "soft spot" of an infant's head is at a normal tension
- Viral HEENT infections including conjunctivitis/pinkeye, ear infections, sore throats and simple colds are very common in childhood, so attention is routinely turned to these areas
- The oral cavity may be both inspected and palpated to assess for a normal sucking reflex as well as teething

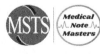

Respiratory exam:

- Respiratory complaints such as cough and wheeze are frequent in the pediatric population, and since this could represent a dangerous illness, reassuring pertinent negative findings should be documented
- Stridor – a high-pitched breathing noise associated with a viral illness known as croup
- Retractions – a child's flexible chest wall may show retractions around the ribs or clavicles where increased pressure changes "suck in" the soft tissues

Neurological exam:

- Mental status is appropriate for age –this statement is often used instead of "alert and oriented"
- Ambulation appropriate for age
- Child reaches for stimulus –simple test for eye/hand coordination

Musculoskeletal exam:

- MAE (moving all extremities) – since some children may not be able to localize pain, or follow commands regarding strength or ROM, the observation that the child is moving all extremities freely might be used

Other exam points:

- Special attention may be paid to the diaper area for rashes or unclear genitourinary complaints
- Rashes are quite common chief complaints, or may be seen in association with other systemic illness like viruses, so include a skin exam
- Children may not be able to verbalize tenderness, rather, they may cry or withdraw from the provider, so document the behavior(s) observed
- Some injuries or behaviors may raise suspicion for child abuse or neglect. In those cases, documentation of pertinent positives and negatives will be even more extensive than usual, often with photographs. Physicians are mandated reporters for suspected abuse.
- The full exam may be limited by the child crying, not cooperating with the provider or other behaviors. As always, document any limitations.

Exam Documentation Examples:

General Appearance- Normal in no acute distress.Clothed exam.

HEENT-Head, NC/AT. Eyes,sclera anicteric, conjunctiva pink, PERRLA. Ears,TM's normal bilaterally. Nose, WNL. Throat,buccal mucosa moist, pharynx beneign.

Neck-No cervical lymphadenopathy, no thyroid enlargement.

Back-No costovertebral angle or vertebral tenderness.

Lungs-good inspiratory effort, clear to auscultation. No rales, rhonchi, wheezes.

Breasts.not performed.

Cardiac-regular rate, no murmurs or gallops heard.

Abdomen-soft, nontender, normoactive bowel sounds in all four quadrants, no HSM. no bruits. No rebound.

Pelvic exam-not performed.

Extremities-no cyanosis clubbing or edema.

Pulses-femoral, dorsalis pedis, and posterior tibialis pulses two plus and equal.

Skin-no abnormal lesions seen at this time.

Neuro-the patient is alert, cooperative, oriented times three. Cranial nerves 2 through 12 grossly intact. Motor and sensation grossly intact. Deep tendon reflexes two plus and equal bilaterally.

VS: bp 124/86, HR 99 RR 22 sat 98% RA T 99.0F

General: awake, alert, sitting upright, unable to carry conversation in full sentences but no distress.

HEENT: NC AT. MMM. Conjunctiva well-perfused. Voice raspy and hoarse.

Neck: full ROM, no LAD

Respiratory: diffuse expiratory wheeze with prolonged expiratory phase, mildly increased respiratory effort. No retractions.

Cardiovascular: RRR S1 S2 wnl, no murmur

Abdomen: deferred

Neuro: ambulatory, facial and extremity movements symmetric

Skin: warm and dry

Re-examination after albuterol nebulization: mild scattered fine expiratory wheeze, normalization of respiratory effort. Sats 99% RA.

Exam	Findings	Details
Constitutional	*	Overall appearance - obese.
Respiratory	Normal	Inspection - Normal. Auscultation - Normal. Effort - Normal.
Cardiovascular	Normal	Regular rate and rhythm. No murmurs, gallops, or rubs.
Musculoskeletal	Comments	No tenderness of lumbar spinous processes, paraspinal muscles, or gluteal muscles b/l. Tenderness over R greater trochanteric bursa. No tenderness of IT band. 5/5 strength lower extremities. 1/4 DTR lower extremities. Difficult to assess hip ROM d/t pain. Pain in all directions with flexion, external rotation, and internal rotation of R hip. Negative straight leg test b/l.
Neurological	Normal	Memory - Normal.
Psychiatric	Normal	Orientation - Oriented to time, place, person & situation. Appropriate mood and affect.

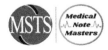

End of Chapter Quiz

1. Which abnormal lung sound is also known as crackles?
   a. Rales
   b. Rhonchi
   c. Wheezing
   d. Sputum
2. Which grade denotes a normal pulse strength?
   a. 1+
   b. 2+
   c. 3+
   d. 4+
3. A rapid heartrate is known as what?
   a. Tachypnea
   b. Tachycardia
   c. Bradycardia
   d. Hypoxia
4. Which term is NOT part of the neck exam?
   a. Tenderness
   b. Lymphadenopathy
   c. Cerumen
   d. Thyromegaly
5. Edema refers to redness surrounding an injury.
   a. True
   b. False
6. The physical exam generally includes:
   a. Inspection
   b. Auscultation
   c. Palpation
   d. All of the above
7. Symptoms are often included in the physical exam.
   a. True
   b. False

Answers: 1. A 2. B 3. B 4. C 5. B 6. D 7. B

5. Objective Sections: Clinical Course, Results, A&P

Clinical Course

The Clinical Course outlines updates and progress that occur after the initial history and physical exam. A Clinical Course should be included any time that tests, consultations, therapies and re-evaluations are performed during the visit to document the timeline of when results returned and how the patient responded to treatments. The intent is to demonstrate the **chronology** of the patient's clinical course, not lengthy descriptions or interpretations that are documented elsewhere.

This section is not always necessary in the clinic, since in-office therapies are not as frequent, and labs and X-rays are usually performed at a separate site. However, some clinics have in-house imaging and labs so that the patient is sent to another

area briefly and returns to get the results. In this case, the results can be documented within the same visit. Aptly named, point-of-care (POC) tests are performed in-clinic with simple methods that provide immediate results, without requiring a formal lab analysis. Urine dipsticks, urine pregnancy tests, fingerstick glucose results, and POC INR are a few examples, which return during the patient visit and should be included in today's note.

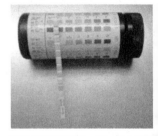

Figure 5.1: POC urine dipstick

Below are a few relatively simple Clinical Course examples:

Clinical Course: TIME patient examined, R wrist XR ordered
TIME XR obtained
TIME XR results return. Interpretation: no fracture
TIME patient advised of results, discharged home with splint

Clinical Course: TIME patient roomed in ER8, seen and examined
TIME fingerstick BS returns 45. D50 ordered.
TIME pt re-examined, mental status normalized. BS 75.

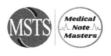

Clinical Course: TIME patient examined, R knee XR and Toradol ordered
TIME patient administered Toradol
TIME XR obtained
TIME Pt returns from XR, no fx
TIME patient advised of results, re-examined. Still having difficulty walking, so immobilizer and crutches fitted
TIME able to ambulate, feeling better, discharged home

In the ED, the Clinical Course or ED Course is usually essential documentation since most visits involve labs, imaging, therapies, consultations, and re-evaluations. The physician's thought process evolves as workup results return, as the patient responds or does not respond to treatments, as vital signs change, etc. Remember, if it isn't documented, it didn't happen, and if the scribe is not paying attention, then critical items of the clinical course may be missed. The adept scribe stays on top of the Clinical Course as it evolves. If updates are documented in real-time, the EHR can often simplify the process because it will pull in the most recent set of vitals, timestamp entries, etc.

Below are more complex examples of two clinical courses for chest pain. Note that the focus is on the timing and sequence of events, leaving the details to other sections of the note. The EKG interpretation and bedside US would have separate procedure notes documented, the discussion with the cardiologist would be summarized in the CDM, and results like the chest XR would have more detail in the results review.

Clinical Course: TIME patient seen and examined
TIME iv inserted, placed on 2L O2 NC
TIME 12-lead EKG obtained, nonacute
TIME patient administered 324mg ASA
TIME request to EMS for transport
TIME ntg SL given q5" x 3
TIME patient is pain-free
TIME VS recheck: HR 85, bp 145/95, sats 99% on 2L NC
TIME pt reports feeling lightheaded
TIME EKG repeated, unchanged
TIME HR 72, bp 130/72, NSR.
TIME d/w patient and wife, consent to transfer
TIME d/w Dr. Brown at El Dorado ER

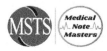

TIME patient departs urgent care

ED Course: TIME patient arrives by ambulance, one iv in place

TIME patient examined, piv placed, monitor, O2 per NC

TIME cardiac monitor shows atrial fibrillation @95bpm

TIME 12-lead EKG obtained + STEMI

TIME Level 1 Cardiac alert called, orders placed; cardiology paged

TIME Patient administered 5 mg metoprolol iv q5" x 3

TIME bedside US performed, no effusion

TIME pCXR performed. Pt pain-free.

TIME VS recheck: HR 85, bp 145/95, sats 99% on 2L NC, afib

TIME HR 72, bp 130/70 after metoprolol. Remains in afib.

TIME Cardiologist paged again

TIME labs return, troponin negative. pCXR negative.

In these examples, the event timeline is crucial for patient care and some are tracked as quality metrics. While the typical ED Course is not often going to be as complicated as for chest pain, the concept is the same for simple visits.

Results Review

Most EHRs can pull in results from today's visit, as well as previous results, by clicking on a particular button or typing a macro that links to the result. The way the EHR pulls in the raw results, however, may be long and messy, taking up pages of space, so some providers prefer to document that the raw results were reviewed and only write out the interpretation. **Every** test that was ordered should be addressed, either with an interpretation or with an indication that the test result is pending. If it isn't documented, it didn't happen. For example:

Results: CBC, BMP, UA results were reviewed and unremarkable. HBA1c results <7 and indicate good control over the last 3 months.

Results: CT head per radiology reveals a suprasellar subarachnoid cyst, details in the radiologist report

Imaging: pCXR personally interpreted, no acute findings, central line in good position, no pneumothorax

Labs: UA c/w contamination, so C&S ordered and pending. UPT neg. Wet prep neg. GC/chlam pending.

Results: CBC reviewed, Hb low today, but at baseline.

	date	result	Normal range
Hemoglobin	8/1/16	12.6	12.1 to 15.5 milligrams per deciliter
Hemoglobin	9/16/17	11.8	12.1 to 15.5 milligrams per deciliter
Hemoglobin	8/15/18	11.4	12.1 to 15.5 milligrams per deciliter
Hemoglobin	3/12/19	11.9	12.1 to 15.5 milligrams per deciliter

Results review: CBC, UA neg. Creatinine wnl. CT chest with contrast: no PE per radiology phone call, official report pending

Results: CBC, BMP, UA results were reviewed. CBC and UA wnl. Serial creatinine results per EHR indicate a significant increase today.

	Date	Result	Reference Range
Creatinine	8/1/16	0.96	0.84 to 1.21 milligrams per deciliter
Creatinine	9/16/17	1.12	0.84 to 1.21 milligrams per deciliter
Creatinine	8/15/18	1.08	0.84 to 1.21 milligrams per deciliter
Creatinine	3/12/19	1.85	0.84 to 1.21 milligrams per deciliter

The Assessment and Plan (A&P)

Finally, the note gets to the point.

This is the culmination of the note, the very reason that the history and physical were performed and the conclusion that the physician drew after analyzing all of the available information. In fact, the A&P is so important that some healthcare providers are moving to an "APSO" note so that the A&P is first and foremost. Traditionally, the assessment and plan are relatively separate elements of the SOAP format, but they may be combined, depending on physician preference and the number of issues addressed at the visit.

A patient presenting with a sore throat may have a relatively simple A&P, but a complex patient with high blood pressure, diabetes, and acute dizziness will need the A&P split up to address all of the patient's issues. If you are listening attentively while the provider interacts with the patient, you should be able to write most of the assessment and plan, because the physician typically

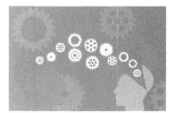

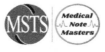

discusses results, diagnosis, and plan with the patient. You will want to change any "layman's" terms that the provider uses with the patient and use a more medical term, but otherwise, remember that anything the provider discusses should be documented. Nonetheless, unless you are a mind-reader, the provider will need to review what you have written in the A&P carefully and likely add additional details based on his/her unspoken insights before signing the note.

Clinical Decision Making (CDM) or Medical Decision Making (MDM)

This section often starts off the A&P for patients with medically complex or risky problems, with a summary of the patient situation and the physician's decision-making process leading up to the actual diagnoses and plan. It is most commonly a paragraph summarizing pertinent items of the history, physical, and workup that led the physician to come to the conclusions and plan. As a scribe, this may be the most challenging portion, since it is a synthesis of many elements that may or may not have been explained to you. In many cases, you can at least get it started based on what you have heard the physician say to the patient or other physicians. If for instance, you hear the physician talking to the hospitalist about why the patient meets admission criteria and cannot be sent home, then this will broadly cover the MDM. With time you may become experienced with the provider's habits, such that you can reasonably draft most of this section before the provider gives you more insight or instruction.

The basic structure is exemplified below, with a backdrop sentence, important elements of the history, elements of the exam, highlights of the workup, diagnoses considered, the assessment, and a summary of the plan. A simple ear infection might not require a long CDM, but chest pain or shortness of breath represent chief complaints with potentially dangerous consequences, so documentation should reflect that risk.

> Julie is a 33 y/o known migraineur who presents with acute on chronic HA. She reports her symptoms are exactly like previous, she required ER visit due to lack of medication at home. She already took 800 mg ibuprofen PTA. Neuro exam nonfocal. After Zofran and SQ Imitrex, pt allowed to rest and on re-exam she is feeling much better, tolerating po. Considering her history and

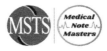

exam, head CT is deferred due to low suspicion for intracranial pathology. We will refill her Imitrex for now, until she is able to see her neurologist.

Patient is a 65 y/o M with risk factors of poorly controlled DM, HTN who presents to the ED with stuttering CP. He was pain-free on arrival but symptom pattern concerning for cardiac etiology. PE unremarkable except for 1+ pitting pretibial edema. He appears well. EKG #1 with nonspecific lateral abnormalities. 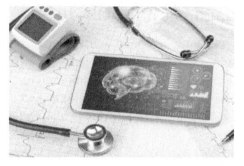 Previous EKG pulled, showing the same lateral flattening. Initial trop neg, but due to stuttering symptoms, timing of troponin to symptoms is unclear. Already took 324 mg ASA just PTA. CXR neg. Pt remained pain-free during stay, VSS. Pt has no previous stress tests or advanced cardiac w/u on file. Due to risk factors and high probability for underlying CAD, he is high risk for discharge home without further workup. d/w hospitalist on call Dr. Adams, who agrees with risk factor assessment and plan for serial troponins and stress test in the morning if appropriate. Pt and wife initially refusing admission, but reluctantly agreed after reviewing risks of d/c.

Pete is a healthy 3 y/o immunized M who presents with URI symptoms and L ear pain x 5 days. He appears well, active, but actively screaming during ear exam. Afebrile, but mom giving Tylenol q4h, sats wnl, lungs clear. Bilat TMs dull and erythematous with cloudy effusion, 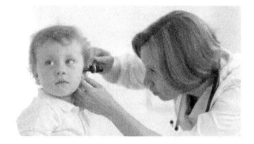 and mild bulging on left. Lack of pt cooperation limited full oropharyngeal exam. Current guidelines indicate antibiotic therapy warranted at this point, we have gone through AOM with pt a few times before and mom is familiar with the 48 h wait-and-see approach from previous visits so she waited for eval. Reviewed previous clinic notes, it has been 5 months since previous amox tx, and his AOM frequency is approaching point for PE tubes. Mom would like to think about it and will call back if she elects ENT referral.

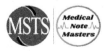

These examples show the synthesis of all other areas of the note, including history, physical, clinical course and results review, without much detail or duplication, since the decision-making elements discussed are covered in detail elsewhere.

Diagnosis and ICD-10

Next, the assessment will be more explicitly made in the form of one or more diagnoses. It may be a long list for patients with multiple chronic medical conditions, or it may be a single diagnosis in a healthy patient presenting with an acute illness or injury. For patients with more than one diagnosis, the provider could elect to split up the CDM and plan for each diagnosis.

The final diagnosis (or diagnoses) is essential for several reasons:
1. Moving forward, it is the most straightforward one-phrase conclusion of the entire visit that other healthcare personnel see.
2. Billing and reimbursement depend upon it.
3. It will likely be carried forward as part of the past medical history or problem list in the EHR.
4. The condition may need to be reported to outside agencies.
5. Quality metrics depend upon it to identify included conditions.

The assessment should be as specific as possible, including the elements below, and a system called ICD-10-CM is used to codify the diagnosis and associated specifics.

- Acute or chronic
- Stable or unstable
- Initial or follow-up visit
- Well-controlled or poorly-controlled
- Laterality/location (when applicable)
- Traumatic or non-traumatic

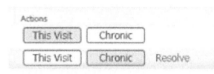

ICD-10, which stands for the International Classification of Disease 10th edition, is a six-digit code attached to diagnoses. This coding system makes it simpler for health care establishments, insurance companies, and regulatory agencies to analyze and compile patient data. The diagnosis may be in the note as free text as well, but entering the diagnosis as **discrete codable** data in the EHR is more valuable since it appears in multiple other areas of the chart as the final conclusion of the visit. In some cases, this data field might be a pick-list of options, or in most cases, there is a smart field whereby you type in the first few letters, and the system provides a list of matches from which to choose (similar to when you begin typing a few letters into an internet search engine). The example below begins with typing

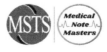

"cellulitis" and then additional specifics can be selected. After selecting the closest match, other specifics can be entered such as acute or chronic.

		L03.011	Cellulitis of right finger
Laterality (3)	▼	L03.012	Cellulitis of left finger
☐ Right		L03.019	Cellulitis of unspecified finger
☐ Left		L03.031	Cellulitis of right toe
☐ Unspecified		L03.032	Cellulitis of left toe
		L03.039	Cellulitis of unspecified toe
Disease process (15)	▶	L03.111	Cellulitis of right axilla
Site (31)	▶	L03.112	Cellulitis of left axilla
		L03.113	Cellulitis of right upper limb
Time Course (2)	▼	L03.114	Cellulitis of left upper limb
☐ Acute		L03.115	Cellulitis of right lower limb
☐ Chronic		L03.116	Cellulitis of left lower limb

Figure 5.2: Example of cellulitis diagnosis entry options in an EHR

Generally, an objective diagnosis is preferred over a subjective symptom when possible. For instance, "low back strain" is preferred over "low back pain." At times, however, no objective diagnosis is found and a symptom will have to suffice.

Diagnosis				Sort Priority	Visit	Updated
New Problem						
Problem:	Lumbar spine strain				🔍	➕ CodeSearch
Display:	Acute, mild, strain of left quadratus lumborum due to slip/fall on 10/17/13.					
Priority:		🔍 Noted:	10/24/2013 📅	☐ Chronic		
Class:		🔍 Resolved:	📅	☐ Show in MyChart		

Figure 5.3: Example of low back strain diagnosis in an EHR

For some patients, such as those well-known to clinic or those presenting for routine care, the visit conversation may seem relatively casual. In those cases, there may not be a great deal of CDM, and the A&P may simply list the patient's known diagnoses and medications, and brief plans such as refills or dates for future screening exams. In the example below, only a quick question is asked but the documentation reflects the physician's full background thought process. If the patient has a number of chronic medical issues, then each should be included if it was even briefly discussed or if any action is required, such as a medication refill.

Provider: "How are you doing with your cholesterol med?"
Patient: "Fine, same as always"
Provider: "Good. We'll repeat your labs in a year."

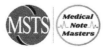

> Diagnosis:
> Hypercholesterolemia
> Refill Lipitor 20 mg po qd. Labs from 8/4 reviewed. LDL at goal and LFTs stable. Next lipid panel 1 year at next annual physical.

Because the diagnosis entry is so crucial, your facility may restrict scribes from entering it (much like allergies). In those situations, the physician will personally select the diagnosis in the designated section of the EHR likely while entering orders for discharge, and then those entries can be pulled into the medical note. You may also be asked to manually type in the assessment details in this section in free text, and then "refresh" so that the link to the EHR entry is updated. For example:

> **A/P:** CHF exacerbation *(free text)*
> 1. Increase Lasix from 20 mg QD to 40 mg QD
> 2. TTE ordered
> 3. Initiate leg compression stockings
> 4. Continue ASA, lisinopril
>
> **Diagnosis**: *(linked from EHR entry after refresh)*
> `Acute on chronic systolic congestive heart failure I50.23`

The complexity of the CDM and associated diagnoses will vary between patients and tends to fall into a few categories.
1. Routine visit, no complaints
2. Routine visit with complaints
3. Acute visit for one or more complaints

Below is another EHR diagnosis example, where additional boxes are available to enter specifics. A final consideration when entering diagnoses is whether or not the diagnosis will be visible to the patient. In most EHRs, patients are able to register for a "portal" account, whereby they can see certain elements of the chart. In some instances, it isn't advisable to release the diagnosis to the patient immediately so there may be a checkbox as pictured below or in Figure 5.3 "Show in MyChart."

Diagnoses

☑ 🔒 Complication occurring during pregnancy ▾

Refine the diagnosis of Complication occurring during pregnancy ▾

Trimester: first trimester ▾

ICD-10: O26.91 Pregnancy related conditions, unspecified, first trimester

☐ Include on Patient Reports

Some notes about this diagnosis. ▾

☑ Add to Problem List   Onset: mm/dd/yy   Problem Note: problem note

Figure 5.4: Diagnosis entry example, highlighting patient visibility

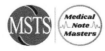

The Plan

The Plan is a summary of the physician's intended care plan after the patient leaves the department, and can range from simple home care to urgent transfer by helicopter. Many portions of the Plan are carried out by parties not present during the visit, so they must rely upon the clarity of the note's written instructions and orders placed. Support staff often facilitate the Plan, calling in appointment requests or filling out paperwork, in adherence to the Plan's documentation. Even small errors can lead at the very least to patient frustration and confusion, but also potentially to serious medical mismanagement. Since the average patient cannot accurately recall all of what was discussed during a physician visit, the documentation can help immensely if the patient calls to ask questions or if misremembering leads to other problems.

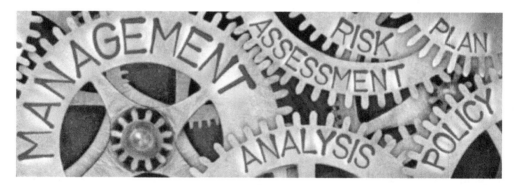

Recall what we learned from the game of "telephone" years ago: each time information is passed from one person to another, the information changes. Similarly, each time the patient passes from one venue to another, there is risk to patient care, so clear and concise documentation reduces that risk.

While the Plan can vary in complexity, some general rules apply as outlined below, with several documentation examples.

1. Write down all elements of the plan discussed, even if it seems obvious or common sense. Include any instruction sheets that were supplied.

   - Rest and avoid strenuous activities for 2-3 days
   - Parents will give the child Tylenol every 4-6 hours for fever. Continue to encourage fluid intake. Avoid sugary liquids.

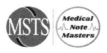

- Patient will remain contagious for the next 2-3 days and will avoid contact with others.
- Patient must thoroughly clean bathroom, kitchen, and other surfaces with disinfectant to avoid bacterial re-infection.
- Do not scratch or itch the rash. Use OTC hydrocortisone cream qid until symptoms resolve, or a maximum of 1 week.
- Unfortunately, the patient did not get his blood drawn before today's appt. He was encouraged to proceed immediately to the lab, and we will call him with the results.

2. Include the anticipated clinical course and recovery time. Giving an anticipated time frame for the duration of symptoms helps set expectations.

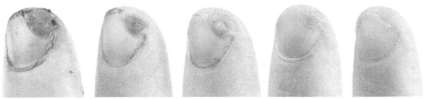

- Wound will likely take 2 weeks to heal. Anticipate oozing will continue for 1-2 more days. Itching is common during healing.
- Symptoms will likely continue for another 24-48 hours, then improve.
- Some delayed or increased musculoskeletal pain is common following an injury. After some possible worsening tomorrow, symptoms should then begin to improve.
- Patient has only had symptoms for 4 hours, without a clear cause, and it is difficult to predict progression. Patient will call us first thing in the morning with an update if symptoms do not resolve.

3. The patient should know when and where to follow-up. "Follow-up as needed" is too vague, since what a provider considers "needed" may differ substantially from what the patient or others might believe. To minimize risk, the provider should specify a time frame as well as possible reasons that the patient should be seen sooner.

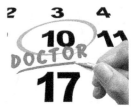

- No specific follow-up is required for the current condition unless symptoms persist longer than expected or new symptoms arise. Patient will return to the clinic in 6 months for routine follow-up.

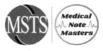

- Patient to see PCP within 2 weeks.
- The patient should keep his psychologist appointment later this week. He has signed a safety contract and agrees to call the suicide helpline or present to the emergency room if he feels unsafe.
- No indications that an orthopedist referral is required at this time. Pt to f/u with PCP to get PT referral and reassessment.

4. Include specifics about any referrals that are to follow, especially if they involve external entities. In some cases, providers in the same healthcare system EHR can send referrals simply through placing an order, and the receiving physician can easily access the patient's EHR information. In other cases, the referral itself is accomplished through a phone call or fax, and the accompanying records must be manually sent. Additionally, consideration for practical matters such as insurance may come into play. For instance, an uninsured patient may need a referral list for low-cost or free dentistry services, or a rural location may not have many referral specialists available. Note that the examples below include the physician's name, department or specialty, referral route, and urgency level.

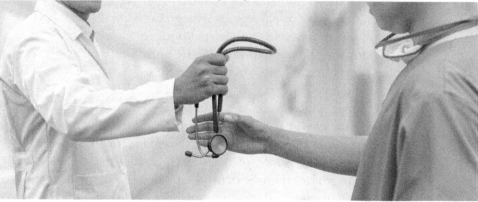

- Referral to dermatology for concerning L ear lesion. Patient wants to see his previous dermatologist Dr. Brown. Due to concern for malignancy, he needs to be seen within 2 weeks. If Dr. Brown's office cannot see him quickly, patient will call us back for assistance.
- Referral to Dr. Jones, GI at St. Louis Healthcare System, for EGD.
    o   Addendum: RN called GI and acquired appt on 10/15 at 10:00 am. Faxed over a copy of today's note and pertinent labs.
- Screening colonoscopy overdue – referral order placed in EHR.

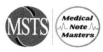

- Will send pt to our office dietician for weight loss. Secure message sent through EHR requesting appt in next 30 days, they will call pt.
- Pt requires urgent ophthalmology evaluation. Called Dr. Globe's office, they will squeeze him in this afternoon. Will transport by private car, pt's wife is driving, he agrees to go straight there. No eating/drinking. Keep eye patch in place.
- Due to patient's age, will refer to urology for urgent evaluation. Spoke with Peachtree Urology on-call, Dr. Silver, who will arrange overbook appointment for patient in the morning.
- Electronic referral sent to Dr. Doe in plastics, non-emergent.
- Patient is changing healthcare systems due to insurance. She will ask for ROI form at the front desk so that we can send her records.
- The patient's case was discussed with Dr. Smith ob/gyn. Orders placed for repeat quant beta, lab slip given to patient to be drawn on 10/15. Dr. Smith's office will call patient to make appointment. Pt will call us back if she doesn't hear from them tomorrow.

5. Include orders, including prescriptions, that are placed for the future. Like referrals, the rationale should be apparent regarding the indication and urgency of the order. Routine prescriptions may be ordered in the EHR, and will be sent electronically to the patient's preferred pharmacy (if entered in the EHR). Often a paper prescription is unnecessary, except for controlled substances. Prescriptions 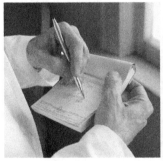 written on paper or called in still need to be entered into the medical record, and the provider should denote that when placing the order. Most EHRs allow for a macro or other shortcut keystroke to be typed in the note that will pull in medication and imaging orders placed during the encounter.

- Refills of all home meds sent via eRx as documented in EHR
- Agreed to refill Vicodin only once more. Rx database checked, results as expected. Called into Walgreens #30.
- Patient given rx for Keflex and location of local 24-hour pharmacy.
- RUQ US ordered to United Radiology to evaluate abnormal labs. Pt given radiology slip and prep sheet.
- Initial vaccine dose given today in clinic. Repeat inoculation at day 7 and day 21 ordered, to be administered at nurse-only visits.

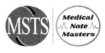

6. Work/school notes are commonly needed, and can be completed using EHR-supplied templates or on paper. Some employers require employees to get a note if they have missed a certain number of days of work, or if any

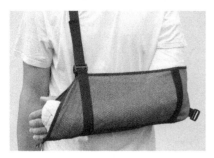

activity restrictions are involved. All worker's compensation-related visits require a work note, which is often quite specific regarding what activities are allowed. The physician and support staff may collaborate to complete paperwork and scan into the EHR, but the Plan should include at least the essential elements of the activity restrictions and/or refer to the specifics of the work note.

Medications

Precise recording of pre-visit, during-visit and post-visit medications is called medication reconciliation, and it is a process intended to reduce medication errors. It begins by assessing all of the patient's current medications when the patient arrives, usually by intake staff then confirmed by the provider. Hence, during the visit, an accurate list is on record to inform the physician's medication ordering decisions. Upon discharge, again the list is reviewed in light of what medications will be added, continued, or stopped. The formal process of medication reconciliation is required during transitions of care such as an admission or transfer, but in general the concept is important for patient safety in all venues. A skilled scribe can be of great assistance in this process, through searching the EHR for missing information, and documenting the medication changes clearly in the Plan. The term "polypharmacy" applies to patients taking multiple daily medications, and can have substantial ramifications regarding interactions and side effects. Roughly 30% of older patients are taking five or more daily medications, and patients often experience confusion regarding which medications they are to take,

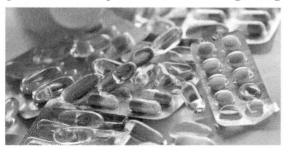

and for what purpose. Thus, each diagnosis and medication should be spelled out in the Plan, such that there is no ambiguity as to which medications are kept the same, changed, or stopped, and often the patient is provided a printout of their medication list for reference.

Examples

In cases of a single diagnosis, the assessment and plan can be in separate sections of the note. When multiple diagnoses are in play, the A&P may be combined as in the following example for ease of organization.

Assessment/Plan

#	Detail Type	Description
1.	Assessment	Essential hypertension (I10), Chronic.
	Patient Plan	BP is 136/84 today in office
		RESTART Lisinopril 10mg daily
		Keep good hydration, avoid adding salt to diet
		Continue w current diet, exercise, and weight loss
		Advised to check BP at home and call if BP is elevated
2.	Assessment	Obesity (BMI 30-39.9) (E66.9), Active.
	Patient Plan	Encouraged to continue w current weight loss
		Increase veggies, salads, greens. Reduce carb and sugar intake
		Continue w regular exercise
3.	Assessment	Elevated liver enzymes (R74.8), Active.
	Patient Plan	Hx of Hep C infection
		Checking labs today
		Reassess after results
	Plan Orders	GGT to be performed.
4.	Assessment	Hx of hepatitis C (Z86.19), Historical.
	Patient Plan	Checking liver enzymes today
		Reassess after results
	Plan Orders	Comp. Metabolic Panel (14) to be performed.
5.	Assessment	Needs flu shot (Z23), Active.
	Patient Plan	Flu shot given
	Plan Orders	Regular Flu - .5ml dose, preservative free, 2020-2021 Status: Administered.
6.	Assessment	Exposure to COVID-19 virus (Z20.828).
	Impression	Pt indirectly exposed at work, pt thinks he had COVID in 02/2020 after wife traveled back from Australia
	Patient Plan	COVID ab test ordered
	Plan Orders	SAR-COV-2 IGG to be performed.

Figure 5.5: Example A&P documentation in an EHR

Below is an HPI from an annual physical exam with a corresponding combined assessment and plan (we are omitting the physical exam for brevity). In this case, separating the assessment and plan makes the most sense because there were multiple issues addressed, and the corresponding plan is adjacent.

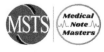

HPI: Bobbi Evans is a 58-year-old female who presents today for an annual physical exam. She has lost 10 lbs recently, about 1 lb per week, and is very happy about this. She achieved weight loss by increasing activity and reducing calories. Her blood pressure has improved and is now averaging 126/81 when she checks it at home.

She has sharp right heel pain that is worst right after she gets out of bed in the morning and when she walks after sitting for a few hours. As she moves around throughout the day, it improves.

She is on methotrexate for psoriasis, which gives her significant nausea, so she would like to discontinue it. Her dermatologist is trying to get it entirely resolved, but she is OK with not achieving completely clear skin. Dermatology also monitors labs for methotrexate.

HEALTHCARE MAINTENANCE: She gets her eyes checked every 1-2 years, and she wears glasses for driving. Dental care is up to date, and she goes every 6-12 months. Immunizations: Tdap in 2015, seasonal influenza 1 year ago.
Screenings: mammogram 2017, normal. Pap 2017 normal, no previous abnormal. Colonoscopy 2019, one polyp removed, next recommended 2024 per GI.

RESULTS: previous labs from 1/20/20 were reviewed, and her cholesterol is at goal. Glucose was not elevated.

ASSESSMENT AND PLAN:

1. Adult physical exam
   a. Cardiovascular risk: blood pressure and cholesterol are at goal. BP was slightly elevated last year but now WNL.
   b. Recent weight loss, intentional, with good results, BMI is now at goal.
   c. Pap and colon cancer screening up-to-date
   d. Influenza immunization given today

2. Encounter for screening for malignant neoplasm of breast
   a. Pt of average risk. Screening mammogram ordered

3. Plantar fasciitis, acute

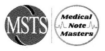

   a. R heel pain is consistent with plantar fasciitis based on history and physical.
   b. Xray deferred
   c. We discussed that both stretches and heel inserts could help with the pain. Stretches are especially helpful after inactivity.

  4. Psoriasis, chronic - she follows closely with derm for this and feels it is under control. No worrisome lesions seen on exam. She has not considered phototherapy yet, but that might be a good option to discuss with derm, given that she would like to discontinue methotrexate.

Below is an HPI from an ER visit with a corresponding combined assessment and plan (we are omitting other sections for brevity). In this case, the diagnoses were listed separately from the MDM and A&P as a style choice, but in reality the EHR largely dictates note formatting, so focus on the content for training purposes.

HPI: Bobbi Harris is a 23 y/o F primigravida who presents to the ER with a 2 d h/o vomiting. Symptoms began gradually maybe a few weeks ago, with just mild intermittent nausea and a "sour stomach," then 2 d PTA she awakened with more overt nausea and vomited breakfast. N/v continued to worsen, and she hasn't been able to keep anything down today. This morning she attempted a nausea "tea" that her friend gave her, but it didn't help and sort of made her dizzy. Denies abd pain, hematemesis, recent travel, unusual food intake, sick contacts, diarrhea.

She reports recent dx of pregnancy. She saw OB 3 d ago for pregnancy confirmation, had a dating US in the office and was told due date was 5/17. She denies pelvic pain, vaginal bleeding or discharge.

ED Course:
1900 pt roomed in 12 and initial hx and physical performed. IV established, IVF ordered. CBC, CMP, UA/UPT ordered. Zofran 4 mg IVP ordered.
1920 HR 98. Bp stable 115/80.
1945 pt feeling better after Zofran. Able to sip some ice water.
2000 HR 86. Labs return, d/w pt glucose level. Able to give urine sample.
2020 HR 88. UA neg ketones, neg glucose, neg protein. UPT pos.
2045 pt feeling much improved. Finished ice water, feels ready for home.

RESULTS: CBC wnl. CMP glucose 148. Utox +THC.

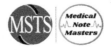

CDM:

23 y/o G1 @ 9wk2d, confirmed IUP with n/v and borderline glucose. Pt is feeling improved after 2L NS and Zofran. Now tolerating po and voices readiness for d/c home. Advised of the elevated glucose level, she denies previous h/o DM although she has a long h/o morbid obesity and multiple family members have type 2 DM. Advised she will likely need a GTT to further investigate. Her previous prenatal visit 9/22 was reviewed and unremarkable, although the urine results were not entered into the EHR. UA today + increased specific gravity, o/w neg. Discussed w/pt +THC in urine, and she admits that the tea contained cannabis, intended to help with nausea. Advised to d/c all cannabis use during pregnancy, and continue to abstain from EtOH and other drugs. She should consult OB before taking OTC meds or supplements, since many are contraindicated in pregnancy.

A&P: Nausea/vomiting and hyperglycemia in early pregnancy
1. VS wnl, no signs of significant dehydration on labs
2. Tolerating PO, good candidate for outpt tx w/antiemetics
3. Rx Zofran ODT 4 mg q4h prn, #30
4. Attempt frequent, small, bland intake. Focus on fluids. Given nausea and vomiting in pregnancy handout.
5. Advised of signs of dehydration, such as reduced urine output
6. Secure message sent to Dr. Infante's office for f/u in the next 3-5 days
7. Return to ED if unable to keep down fluids, lightheadedness, bleeding, abd pain or other concerning symptoms
8. Confirmed IUP by previous US, no symptoms to suggest threatened Ab
9. Continue prenatal vitamin, but high iron content can tend to cause nausea, consider switch to different formulation in d/w her OB

Diagnoses:
abnormal glucose in pregnancy O99.810
Vomiting in pregnancy O21.9
Cannabis misuse F12.10

Note Changes and Addenda

Ideally, the note is finalized at the time of the visit, the provider signs it shortly thereafter, and no changes need to be made later. Different EHRs have different terms for saving, sharing, finalizing, and signing the note, that you will need to learn on your first day so that you click the correct button to indicate you are finished

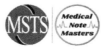

with your portion of the documentation. In most cases, after the note is completed, it CANNOT be easily changed, so the note should be closely double-checked for accuracy before finishing it out. What if there are substantial errors? Suppose you clicked on the wrong patient in the schedule and documented the entire note under the wrong patient's name (which is actually not that unusual). It clearly needs to be fixed, but it's not as simple as deleting the incorrect note and copying it onto a new patient. Once something is entered into the 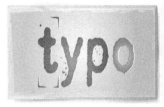 record, it cannot be truly deleted, because the note is a legally signed document. Instead, the erroneous entries are marked as "in error" and crossed-out, then new information is entered. The EHR may have the option to "modify" or open an old note for editing, but the previous documentation is archived to prevent nefarious modification of past entries if medical errors occur or a malpractice case is filed.

Addenda, on the other hand, can be quite ordinary, since patient care issues are often changing. Let's say a patient is seen in the morning, prescribed medication X, but later goes to the pharmacy and finds it is too expensive. In the afternoon, the nurse asks if the provider can change it to something else, but the earlier note has already been signed. Adding an addendum to the note indicating the medication change would be appropriate documentation.

Other follow-up issues like calling patients back with results can be documented via an addendum or by making a new telephone follow-up note. Many clinical practices have a process to review labs and other results that come back after the patient has left. These may 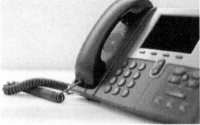 be handled mainly by staff and reviewed by the physician only when an abnormal result appears, or other actions need to be taken. For instance, a patient had a negative rapid strep test and was sent home with symptomatic care only. Then two days later, the culture result returns positive, so the patient now needs antibiotics. The physician will be alerted with this result, will decide upon an antibiotic, and may call back the patient or have staff do so, but the documentation in the chart must reflect that follow-up was successfully completed. Remember the golden rule– if it isn't documented, it didn't happen. If the physician assumes the nurse will take care of it – it didn't happen. If the nurse calls in a prescription and doesn't document it in the EHR – it still "didn't happen." If a message is left for the patient, and no one returns the call – it really didn't happen.

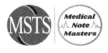

Communication with Other Providers

In the EHR era, it is often assumed that other providers can access your note easily; however, it is not always the case. Recall in the HIPAA chapter that different healthcare systems cannot freely access patient information without explicit patient consent, so times arise where the freshly completed note has to be sent elsewhere for continuity of care. In the case of an emergent transfer to the ER or from the ER to another facility, note documentation must be completed very quickly so the receiving facility has all necessary information to care for the patient.

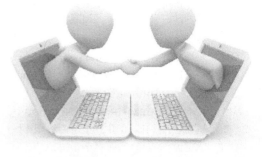

Another example would be a PCP referral to a dermatologist who uses a different EHR, and after the visit, the dermatologist must send the information back to the referring provider. This communication must be accomplished in a HIPAA-compliant manner, preferably through secure EHR messaging. EHRs can generate a clinical summary or a continuity of care document (CCD), which is in a standardized technical format that can be more easily transmitted between EHRs. Encrypted fax or sometimes plain old mailed paper are other options. In any case, the note should specify how the communication was handled.

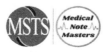

End of Chapter Quiz

1. What should be included in the Clinic/ED course?
   a. Labs, imaging, therapies, consultations, and re-evaluations
   b. Labs, imaging, and therapies
   c. Consultations and re-evaluations
   d. Labs, therapies, and re-evaluations
2. What does ICD stand for?
   a. Important classification of disease
   b. International certification of disease
   c. International classification of disease
   d. Important certification of disease
3. Which of the following should be included in an assessment?
   a. Acute or chronic
   b. Stable or unstable
   c. Well-controlled or poorly-controlled
   d. All of the above
4. When is an addendum a necessary component to the note?
   a. When changes are made to the note before being signed off
   b. When changes are made to the note after being signed off
   c. When changes are made to the note before or after being signed off
   d. Never – you can just edit the note
5. Since providers are able to see results very quickly in the EHR, there is no need to specify that the provider reviewed the results.
   a. True
   b. False
6. A clinic visit should only list 1-2 diagnoses to reduce confusion.
   a. True
   b. False
7. Medication errors are common, so the Plan should specify all medications to be started, continued, or stopped.
   a. True
   b. False

Answers: 1. A 2. C 3. D 4. B 5. B 6. B 7. A

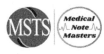

6A. The Primary Care Clinic

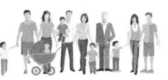

Primary care refers to a group of medical providers that serve as the initial and centralized point of patient care, which typically includes:

- Pediatrics—care for children up until early adulthood
- Internal medicine—focused on adult medicine
- Geriatrics—care for elderly patients
- Family practice—care for patients of all ages, from infants to the elderly
- Obstetrics and gynecology—specialized in women's health, including preventative care and reproductive health (gynecology) and monitoring pregnancy and delivery (obstetrics)

These providers may practice in a hospital or a clinic, but this chapter is directed towards those providers that operate in a clinic. This is called "outpatient" medicine vs. "inpatient" medicine, which refers to the care of patients admitted to a hospital.

For healthy patients, a primary care provider (PCP) may be their only medical provider, but when more specialized care is required, the PCP can refer to a specialist. For example, a patient may present to a PCP with shoulder pain, then begin physical therapy for six weeks. If the patient returns afterward with ongoing shoulder pain, the PCP then may refer the patient to an orthopedic specialist for further evaluation and treatment. The patient may see many specialists at one time or another, but the PCP is the central hub of care (hence *primary* care). Without a primary physician, a patient's care can be fragmented amongst various providers that do not communicate, and care quality suffers.

Most outpatient clinics have a familiar organization and flow. Patients first enter the clinic and are greeted at the registration desk. Here, the patient checks in for the appointment, provides insurance information, and fills out any required forms. Then, a medical assistant (MA/CMA) or nurse will find the patient in the waiting area and bring the patient back to a room for vital signs, to review forms and routine screenings, obtain a brief history ("what brings you in today?"), and verify current medications. The EHR is updated with this information, and the patient is marked as "Ready for Provider" or a similar indicator.

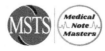

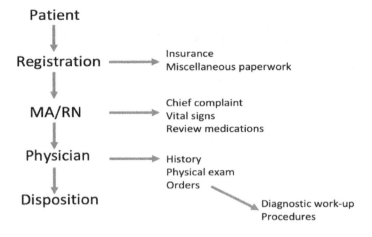

Figure 6.1: Typical patient flow through a clinic

At this point, the provider will take a moment to review the intake and other information to prepare for the encounter, then the provider and scribe will enter the room. As the conversation unfolds, the scribe takes notes and documents all pertinent information either directly into the EHR in the room, or with shorthand notes on paper to be entered into the computer later. The provider may order labs or radiology studies, and depending on the type of clinic, some simple labs and radiology studies may be performed within the clinic or at an outside facility.

For point-of-care and time-sensitive tests, the patient will wait until the results have returned, but in most scenarios, the patient will be notified of the results via phone or secure EHR message after a day or two. The medical note should indicate which tests have been ordered and are pending. Before patients leave the clinic, they are often given a printed visit summary/patient plan generated by the EHR. This "after visit summary" is a document describing the tests performed, medications ordered, immunizations and other medications administered, written recommendations from the provider, and often informational patient handouts for medical conditions.

Your goal as a scribe is to complete every note contemporaneously with the visit, but often some clarification or just additional typing time is required after leaving the room. The provider may go straight to the next patient or take care of miscellaneous tasks such as refill requests and phone calls if there is a gap between appointments. Most of these tasks still require documentation, so the scribe is seldom idle, but if there is still downtime between patients, you can prepare for upcoming appointments by pulling previous notes or results.

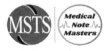

Common Patient Encounters

Patients may present to the clinic for any number of reasons, but a large proportion of the visits fall into easily definable categories that are worth taking the time to understand. Some of these include routine visits like annual physicals, well-child checks, sports physicals, and pre-operative visits. This chapter will describe the purpose of many types of visits and the typical diagnostics performed during each.

Table 6.1: Most frequent reasons for primary care visits

Upper respiratory symptoms, sore throat	Joint or back pain
Blood pressure, cholesterol	Headache
Routine/preventative/well-child	Rash
Diabetes	Depression/anxiety/stress
Medication refill/evaluation	Test results
Pre- and post-op	Abdominal pain

Annual Physicals and Preventative Medicine

Patients new to a particular clinic may have an initial visit aptly named a "new patient visit." These visits are intended for the patient to "establish care" (these are the keywords) with the provider, rather than address an acute complaint like a sore throat. This involves going over the patient's prior medical, surgical, family, and social history, as well as addressing preventative screenings and other healthcare

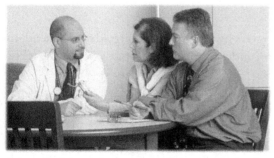

maintenance. Your job as a scribe is to make sure these various details are up to date in the EHR for future visits. The multiple preventative screens will be detailed here because a general knowledge can help write the HPI and the assessment and plan.

Annual visits are commonplace, even for healthy patients, to review preventative care. Some insurers (Medicare PHP, VA) require a yearly visit. The chief complaint might be "Annual Wellness Visit," and patients may or may not have acute issues they would also like to address. From the physician's perspective, these visits allow dedicating time to more thoroughly review healthcare history, screening tests, and disease risk factors.

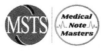

Annual evaluations vary based upon the age and physical sex of the patient, but since most patients do not present for preventative visits until later adulthood, some generalities apply. The top causes of preventable death in the United States consistently remain cardiovascular disease (cardiac and strokes), cancers, and respiratory diseases (such as COPD). They are considered preventable because the underlying disease risk factors of smoking, obesity, hyperlipidemia and hypertension can be prevented and treated. Many cancers can also be prevented through screening exams such as colonoscopies, mammograms and pap smears.

High blood pressure/Hypertension (HTN)

Nearly half of US adults have high blood pressure. Since elevated blood pressure is usually asymptomatic, checking blood pressure at preventative visits can diagnose HTN in its early stages and prevent later complications.

Smoking Cessation

About 16 million Americans live with a smoking-related disease, and tobacco use is the single leading cause of preventable death. It is good practice to cover the 5 A's: Ask all patients about smoking, Advise all smokers to quit, Assess readiness to quit,

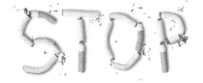

Assist smokers to quit, and Arrange follow-up. Pharmacotherapy is also available, such as nicotine replacement modalities like gum and patches, and the medications varenicline and bupropion.

Geriatric Decline

America's elderly population is rising in number, and alongside, the need for assistance services. Hearing loss can hinder communication, even during clinic visits where it is often documented as HOH (hard-of-hearing). Safety and fall risk are frequent concerns, along with dementia and other memory problems. Activities of Daily Life (ADL) issues like dressing, bathing, cooking, and cleaning can become issues over time, and primary care clinics may need to work closely with the family to facilitate home care or facility placement.

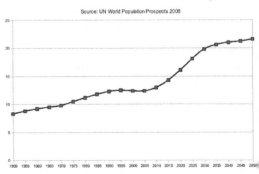

Figure 6.2: Rise in the % of the population >65

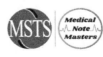

Obesity and Diabetes

The Centers for Disease Control (CDC) estimates that about 40% of Americans are obese, which leads to conditions such as heart disease, stroke, type II diabetes, and certain types of cancer. Adult BMI (body mass index) assessment is an increasingly important quality performance measure, followed by recommendations for lifestyle and dietary modifications. In addition to diabetes, obesity is closely related to some of the most routine clinic visits listed in Table 1, such as joint and back pain, HTN, and depression, so while it is not itself a top clinic diagnosis, it is related to many.

Colon Cancer

Like many cancers, colon cancer is asymptomatic in its early stages so screening exams are required for early diagnosis. The American Cancer Society and the US Preventative Services Task Force (USPSTF) recommend adults between 45 and 75 be screened for colon cancer, but screening may start earlier for patients at higher risk. For average-risk patients, screening might begin with newer assays that can detect worrisome cancer compounds with just a mailed-in stool sample (you may have seen advertisements). A colonoscopy, however, remains the gold standard. The procedure's camera illuminates the colon's interior lining to detect pre-cancerous polyps for removal. If polyps or other abnormalities are seen, the gastroenterologist gives recommendations regarding how frequently colonoscopy should be repeated. When the PCP reviews the report, the findings and recommendations are added to the patient's history and preventative medicine sections of the local EHR.

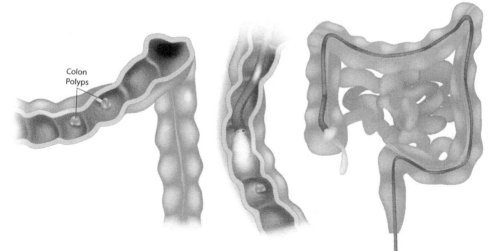

Colon
Polyps

Figure 6.3: Schematic of colonoscopy procedure

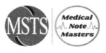

Bone Loss Screening

Although bone loss is most often associated with older females, both men and women experience bone loss with aging. Preventatively, patients may take calcium and vitamin D supplements along with physical exercise to slow the rate of loss.

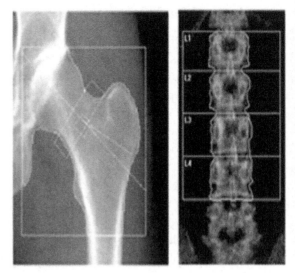

Particularly after menopause, women are at an increased risk of developing the bone-thinning disorders osteopenia and osteoporosis. Natural menopause typically occurs in the late 40s or early 50s, and the associated

Figure 6.4: Areas evaluated for bone density – the femoral neck and the spinal column.

hormone decline increases the rate of bone loss. Screening typically begins at age 65, but hormone decline for other reasons at any age also increases risk, so screening may be initiated earlier in some patients. Aside from sex hormones, other factors increase bone loss including alcohol use, smoking, thyroid disease, chronic inflammation and medications. Thus, men and younger women may be at risk and receive testing earlier.

Dual-Energy X-ray Absorptiometry (DEXA) is one of the most common types of bone density screening tests. The most important result is called the overall T-score, which compares the patient's bone density to what would be expected for a comparable healthy 30-year-old person. The T score can indicate an increased risk of complications such as spinal compression fractures or hip fractures. Calcium and vitamin D remain mainstays, but do not reverse bone loss, so severe cases may be prescribed a bisphosphonate medication that reduces bone breakdown such as alendronate (Fosamax).

Ranges for T-scores include:

T-score of -1.0 to -2.5 is defined as osteopenia ("reduced bone")
T-score of <-2.5 is defined as osteoporosis ("porous bones")

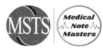

Annual Physicals: Male Organ-Specific

Prostate Disease

Beginning as early as age 45, men may start receiving a prostate (rectal) exam. The prostate gland surrounds the urethra, and enlargement can be associated with urinary symptoms. Benign Prostatic Hypertrophy (BPH), as the name implies, is benign enlargement that occurs in most men as part of aging, as opposed to a malignant enlargement like a tumor. Abnormalities on the physical exam may lead to further testing for cancer, such as ultrasound or a prostate-specific antigen (PSA) blood test. Elevations in the prostate antigen can be associated with BPH and prostate cancer, but it is not a universal screening test because the risks and benefits are not clear. As of 2018, the USPSTF no longer recommends routine PSA screening for males 55-69. Given this, PSA testing may be more likely to be performed in males with a particular indication for testing or under the care of a urologist.

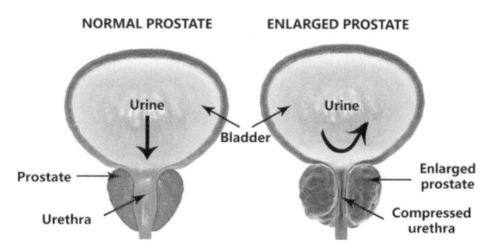

Figure 6.5: Urinary retention associated with an enlarged or inflamed prostate

Testicular Cancer

Younger adult men may be screened for testicular cancer (and hernias) with a genitalia exam. The scrotal exam entails palpation of each testicle to assess for lumps that may indicate testicular cancer, as well as bulges while coughing that may represent an inguinal (groin) hernia. It is performed in men of all ages.

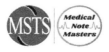

Annual Physicals: Female Organ-Specific

Cervical Cancer Screening

Beginning at age 21, women get cervical exams to screen for cervical cancer. This process involves doing a speculum exam and then swabbing the cervix to collect cells, commonly known as a Pap smear (named after the physician who developed the process). Paps are performed to look for abnormal cells that may indicate cancerous or precancerous changes, called dysplastic cells or cervical dysplasia. Paps are conducted every three years in low-risk women 21-30 years old if no abnormalities are found. After age 30, low-risk women can combine Pap smears with testing for high-risk strains of the human papillomavirus (HPV). HPV is a sexually transmitted virus associated with a majority of cervical cancers, so screening for the presence of HPV can help identify women at higher risk for cervical cancer. Immunization for HPV became available in 2006, making cervical cancer uniquely preventable through immunization. If negative, Pap smears and HPV co-testing only need to be performed every five years. After age 65, women with three negative Pap smears in the past ten years can cease screening Paps. If a Pap smear comes back abnormal at any point, further testing may be required, such as a colposcopy, and testing frequency is increased. Documentation in the record should indicate if a Pap smear is strictly for routine screening purposes or for follow-up of abnormal Paps.

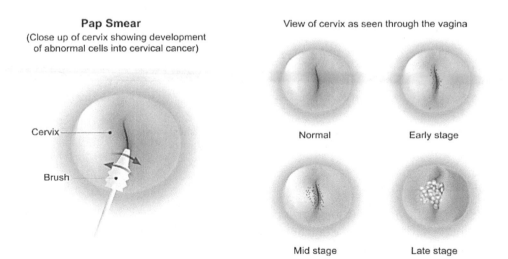

Pap Smear
(Close up of cervix showing development
of abnormal cells into cervical cancer)

View of cervix as seen through the vagina

Cervix

Brush

Normal

Early stage

Mid stage

Late stage

Figure 6.6: The Pap smear and cervical appearance

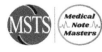

Breast Cancer Screening

Cervical cancer is one of the leading causes of death in women, but breast cancer is the single most deadly cause. Breast cancer screening often begins with breast self-exams, since over half of breast cancers are first detected by a woman or her partner feeling a lump or other abnormality. If a mammogram or other kind of test is done on an asymptomatic patient, it is a *screening* test. If a mammogram is done because of symptoms or exam findings, it is a *diagnostic* test.

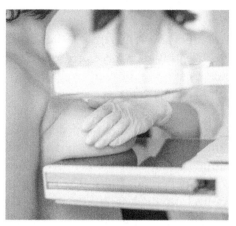

Figure 6.7: Performing a mammogram

Annual or biannual mammograms begin as early as age 30 or as late as age 50. The guidelines for mammogram screening vary depending on the organization, but generally, screening begins at age 40-45 and repeats every 1-2 years if no abnormalities are found. A mammogram uses low-energy x-rays to detect density changes within the breasts, such as a mass, calcification, or abnormally dense breast tissue region. These lumps or masses may be an early sign of breast cancer, and early detection can be lifesaving. If a mammogram comes back with suspicious or abnormal results, the patient will usually undergo additional imaging, an ultrasound or biopsy to understand the abnormality further.

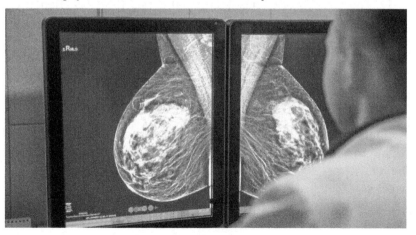

Figure 6.8: Mammogram images

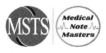

Prenatal Care

Women are carefully monitored throughout pregnancy, through primary care providers, obstetricians, and/or certified nurse midwives (CNM). Some family practice providers focus on obstetrics and care for pregnancy from beginning to end, but most may provide only initial prenatal care before transferring primary responsibility for the pregnancy to an obstetric specialist.

When a woman first suspects she is pregnant, she will often present simply to confirm and officially document pregnancy. Confirmation of pregnancy can be a significant socioeconomic event for some patients, changing insurance and emancipation eligibility. The first prenatal visit is typically scheduled after about 8 weeks from the last menstrual period (LMP). The usual SOAP note format will add ob/gyn histories to the past medical history, and questioning will focus on risk factors for possible pregnancy complications, including previous miscarriages, a dangerous home situation, underlying medical problems, unsafe medications, etc.

The HPI will start with at least the patient's Gravida Para (GP) number. Gravida is the total number of pregnancies and para is the number of births. "A" may be included to count the number of elective + spontaneous abortions. For example: a pregnant patient who has had 1 miscarriage and 2 term live births would have a gravida para number of G4P2A1. The TPAL system is also widely used to further specify Para status, where T= #term births, P= #preterm births, A= #abortions (spontaneous + elective), and L= #living children. The previous example would then be G4P2012. The first day of the last menstrual period (LMP) is often also included in the HPI setup, since it is used to date pregnancy. When possible, it is simplest to review previous notes for this backdrop information. For example:

Maria is a 23 y/o G4P2103 at 10 weeks by LMP 3/6 who presents for…

Table 6.2: Prenatal lab schedule

Weeks along	Labs/Screenings performed
First visit (around 8 weeks or later if patient is unaware of pregnancy)	CBC, blood type, UA, Rubella, syphilis, Pap, GC/chlamydia, HIV, Hep B and C, varicella, +/- sickle cell, +/- TB
18-20 weeks	Ultrasound exam
26-28 weeks	Glucose challenge screening, +/- Rh antibodies, recheck CBC
36-37 weeks	Group B strep test

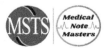

After the initial appointment, the pregnant patient comes in every 4 weeks. At these monthly appointments, maternal weight, fetal heart rate, and growth will be tracked. The patient is likely to start feeling the fetus move at 16-25 weeks, and Gross Fetal Movement (GFM or just FM) is documented. The physical exam will include the fundal height, which is the abdominal level at which the top of the uterus is palpated, as well as grading lower extremity edema. Maternal blood pressure is monitored throughout pregnancy, and especially after 20 weeks, for signs of pre-eclampsia. Pre-eclampsia is a potentially dangerous condition hallmarked by elevated blood pressure as well as kidney and liver problems that requires prompt diagnosis and treatment.

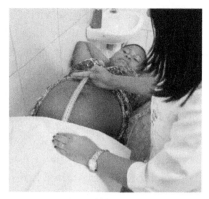

Figure 6.19: Measuring fundal height

Around 28 weeks, the patient begins coming in every 2 weeks. Glucose measurements are taken to evaluate for gestational diabetes, which is as the name implies, diabetes that develops during pregnancy (not pre-existing). High blood sugars affect up to 10% of pregnancies and can lead to several complications including elevated birth weight.

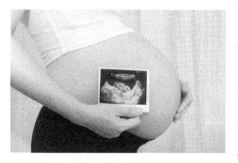

At around 36 weeks, the patient comes in for weekly visits. These visits may include a biophysical profile, which is used to help monitor the baby's health as the due date comes closer. While many patients focus on the due date, only around 5% of women actually deliver on their due date. The initial Estimated Due Date or EDD is calculated based on adding 40 weeks from the first day of the LMP and may be updated after more accurate dating information comes in. Usually "preterm" or "preemie" birth is most concerning for births occurring before 37 weeks. At 39 weeks, the fetus is considered "term" and some pregnancies even last 41 weeks and are "post-term." Throughout this process, the provider and patient will continue to discuss the safest delivery options and plan including birthing location, instructions for what to do when labor begins, etc.

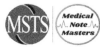

Well Child Checks (WCC)

Much like the preventative visits for adults, children also receive regular check-ups from their PCPs. These visits are called well-child checks (WCC), and they are an essential tool to monitor many aspects of health and development. If concerns ever arise regarding possible child abuse or neglect, healthcare providers are required to report those concerns (termed a "mandated reporter"). Ideally this never arises, but if it does, documentation must be exceptionally detailed, possibly including photos.

Newborns

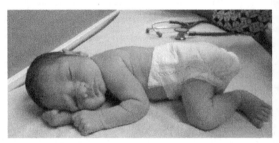

Neonates, or newborn babies, typically require follow up with a physician 2-3 days after leaving the hospital to make sure the baby is feeding adequately, to assess possible jaundice, and to monitor circumcision healing in boys. Birth weight, discharge weight, and possibly Apgar scores from the facility where the infant was born must be in the note, but may not be in the current EHR. APGAR stands for Appearance, Pulse, Grimace, Activity, and Respiratory effort, and lower scores are associated with higher complication rates.

Neonatal weight is closely monitored for several reasons. After birth, up to 10% weight loss is not unusual, but with adequate feeding, the weight should steadily increase. In breast-feeding mothers, quantifying milk intake can be difficult and, at times, a lactation consultant is utilized to assist.

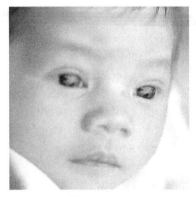

Figure 6.9: Icteric sclera in a neonate (Attribution BY 2.0)

Jaundice is a yellow discoloration of the skin and eyes due to elevated levels of bilirubin, a product of hemoglobin breakdown. While in the womb, bilirubin is processed by the mother's liver. After birth, the baby's liver must start performing this function, and it takes time for the liver to become self-sufficient. Thus, it is not uncommon for newborns to have some degree of jaundice, which can be estimated by the level of yellow color on exam and via lab testing if needed. More severe cases require serial lab measurements and further treatment.

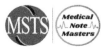

Infants and Toddlers

Well-child checks for young children focus primarily on the child's physical and mental development. The typical appointments occur at 2, 4, 6, 9, 12, 15, 18, and 24 months of age. Growth charts at these visits will track the infant's increase in height and weight compared to other infants of the same age. Growth charts used to be plotted manually on a form such as the one pictured, but now they are typically produced by the EHR. After entering the child's height, weight, or head circumference, the EHR will plot the points on the patient's growth chart and calculate the percentages. Ideally, a child should continue along a growth curve (percentile), and it is worrisome if a patient starts dropping below or rising above their previous percentile from one visit to the next.

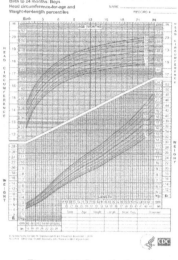

Figure 6.10 Growth chart for boys 0-24 months old

The mental, emotional, and social development of the child is equally important. Together with physical growth, the appropriate development in these categories is called "milestones." The Centers for Disease Control and Prevention (CDC) lists 3-4 milestones at each age, but the exact milestones are unnecessary to memorize. Milestones are tracked because they give providers and guardians opportunities for early intervention when milestones are missed. Milestones are discussed at each WCC, but there are specific screenings recommended at 9, 18, and 30 months so most clinics utilize a standardized questionnaire, such as the Ages and Stages Questionnaire (ASQ). If abnormalities are found, the provider can give recommendations to and refer to specialists if necessary. Autism spectrum disorder screenings also occur at 18 and 24 months.

Table 6.3: Some common milestones in the first five years

Age	Some Common Milestones
2 months	Begins to smile, coos, turns head toward sounds
4 months	Copies some facial expressions, babbles, smiles spontaneously
6 months	Starts recognizing strangers, responds to name, begins to jabber, responds to emotions

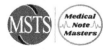

9 months	Afraid of strangers and clings to known adults, copies sounds, points at objects
1 year	Plays peek-a-boo games, uses gestures like waving, can say some words like "mama" and "dada," "cruises" along furniture
18 months	Says several words, points to what is wanted, can follow simple instructions, shows affection
2 years	Knows names of people and body parts, repeats words, finds things, can kick a ball and sort toys
3 years	Takes turns, understands ownership, plays make-believe, can ride a tricycle, can do simple puzzles
4 years	Sings songs, tells stories, hops on one foot, can use scissors
5 years	Aware of gender, can tell the difference between real and pretend, can print letters and numbers, can do a somersault

Table 6.4: Missed milestones

Age	Things to Discuss
2 months	Does not smile at people, respond to loud noises, or watch moving things; can't hold head up
4 months	Does not coo or make sounds, bring things to mouth, or smile at people; has trouble with moving eyes
6 months	Does not reach for things, show affection, or respond to sounds; does not laugh or rollover, is overly stiff or "floppy"
9 months	Does not babble, play games, respond to name, or recognize people; does not sit or bear weight with support
1 year	Does not crawl, stand when supported, or point at things, does not say single words or loses previous skills
18 months	Does not copy others, gain new words, or use at least 6 words, cannot walk, loses previous skills
2 years	Does not use 2-word phrases, walk steadily, or know what to do with everyday objects, loses previous skills
3 years	Drools, falls down often, does not understand simple instructions, does not make eye contact, or want to play with children or toys
4 years	Ignores other children, does not respond to people outside of the family, cannot retell a story, speaks unclearly, loses previous skills
5 years	Limited emotions; extreme behaviors; is withdrawn; cannot do simple tasks like brush teeth or get dressed; loses previous skills

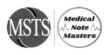

Vaccinations/immunizations are another essential part of well-child checks. The vaccination schedule is quite complicated, and recommendations change from time to time, so memorizing the exact guidelines is not useful. You should, however, be able to recognize and correctly spell immunizations in a medical note, be able to document discussions regarding consent or non-consent for vaccinations, and find the designated section for immunization information in the EHR.

Table 6.5: Common immunizations

Immunization	Disease
Hepatitis A & B	Viral infections affecting the liver
Rotavirus	A common cause of severe diarrhea in children
TDaP	Tetanus, Diphtheria, and acellular Pertussis ("whooping cough"), disease-causing bacteria
HIB	Haemophilus influenza type b, a bacterial cause of meningitis and pneumonia
Inactivated poliovirus (iP)	Polio, a viral infection that can cause paralysis
Influenza	The seasonal flu virus, many formulations available
Pneumococcal (Prevnar-13, Pneumovax)	Streptococcus pneumoniae, a bacterium causing pneumonia and other respiratory ailments
MMR	Measles, Mumps, Rubella, disease-causing viruses
Varicella (Shingrix, Zostavax)	Varicella zoster virus, the cause of chicken pox and shingles

Table 6.6: Immunization schedule

Age	Immunizations
2 months	Rotavirus; Haemophilus Influenzae Type B (HIB); Pneumococcal; Diphtheria, Tetanus, Pertussis (DTaP); Polio (IPV); Hepatitis B (HBV)
4 months	Rotavirus; Haemophilus Influenzae Type B (HIB); Pneumococcal; Diphtheria, Tetanus, Pertussis (DTaP); Polio (IPV); Hepatitis B (HBV)
6 months	Rotavirus; Pneumococcal; Diphtheria, Tetanus, Pertussis (DTaP); Polio (IPV); Hepatitis B (HBV); Influenza (seasonal)
9 months	Influenza

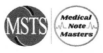

12 months	Measles, Mumps, Rubella (MMR); Chickenpox (Varicella); Hepatitis A; Influenza (seasonal)
15 months	Haemophilus Influenzae Type B (HIB); Pneumococcal; Diphtheria, Tetanus, Pertussis (DTaP); Influenza (seasonal)
18 months	Hepatitis A; Influenza (seasonal)
2 years	Lead (lab); Influenza (seasonal)
2.5 - 3 years	Influenza
4 or 5 years	Diphtheria, Tetanus, Pertussis (DTaP); Polio (IPV); Measles, Mumps, Rubella (MMR); Chickenpox (Varicella); Influenza
6 - 10 years	Influenza
11 years	Diphtheria, Tetanus, Pertussis (Tdap); Meningococcal (MCV); Human Papillomavirus (HPV); Influenza
12 – 15 years	Influenza, COVID
16 years	Meningococcal (MCV); Influenza
17 years	Influenza
18 years	Diphtheria, Tetanus, Pertussis (Tdap); Influenza
19 years +	Influenza

Adolescents

As children continue to get older, the topics discussed at their well-child checks will change. Instead of milestones, a provider may instead ask about school performance as an indicator of development. Teachers or counselors may contribute information, including scoliosis screening, to be incorporated into the note. Concerns about substance abuse, social media, or ill-advised sexual activities may arise which necessitate further recommendations and referrals.

Another change that is apparent as children grow older is the change in relationship with the provider. More and more of the HPI will come from the patients themselves instead of just the guardians. Thus, the provider and patient will start to form an independent relationship and at some point, the visit can partially occur without a guardian in the room. Forging a trusting relationship allows the patient to more freely express concerns and be truthful about sensitive topics such as sexual activity. Information disclosed can generally be kept in confidence, so long as doing so would not represent a tangible danger to the patient or others. As always, healthcare providers are mandated reporters of abuse and neglect for minors.

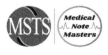

The progression of puberty hallmarks adolescence, often documented by items on the Tanner scale, as shown in the following table.

Tanner Stage	Males	Females
Stage 1: Prepubescent	• No pubic hair • Bone age younger than 12 years	• No pubic hair • No breast development • Bone age younger than 11 years
Stage II	• Minimal pubic hair • Bone age younger than 12 years	• Minimal pubic hair • Breast buds • Bone age younger than 11 years
Stage III: Pubescent	• Pubic hair over penis • Voice changes • Bone age of 13 to 14 years	• Pubic hair on mons • Enlargement of breasts • Axillary hair • Bone age of 12 to 13 years
Stage IV	• Adult pubic hair • Axillary hair • Bone age of 13 to 14 years	• Adult pubic hair • Areola enlargement • Bone age of 12 to 13 years
Stage V: Postpubescent	• As adult • Bone age of 14 to 16 years	• As adult • Bone age of 13 to 14 years

Sports physicals are typically performed for teenagers before participating in a contact sport. Often these teenagers are high-school-aged and generally healthy, and therefore, seldom require workup. The physician will perform a full physical exam during this encounter but with particular attention to heart murmurs and possible hernias. A rare condition called hypertrophic cardiomyopathy can cause sudden death in young persons, and may be detectable through hearing a heart murmur.

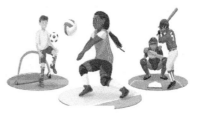

Pre-Operative (Pre-Op) Visits

If a patient has a surgical procedure planned, the surgeon typically requests a pre-operative visit through primary care to assess medical risks. The tests performed during this visit will depend on the patient's age, medical history, and the extent of the procedure. Patients above a certain age or with a prior cardiac history will have an EKG. A CBC or blood type will be ordered if significant blood loss is expected in a riskier procedure. Other common lab tests include UA, UPT, renal function, and blood clotting assessments like INR, which as always, require interpretation.

Scribes should carefully document all instructions the patient was given since proper preparation for surgery prevents complications. Pausing certain medications like blood thinners is commonly required.

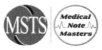

6. The Primary Care Clinic

Pre-operative visits should list any conditions that the surgeon or anesthesiologist should know. Documentation should include the diagnosis for which the surgery is sought as well as the pre-op encounter. For example, if a patient has a right total knee replacement planned, then M17. 11 Unilateral primary osteoarthritis, right knee and Z01.818 Encounter for preprocedural examination would both be listed. You should also include other pertinent conditions such as hypertension or diabetes in your note, so the surgical team has the information required to assess the risks and benefits. If the surgeon uses a different EHR, the note may be manually sent and the note should indicate the recipient(s). Below is an example of a pre-op history entry in an EHR, with corresponding assessment and plan.

Commit **Pre-Operative Visit** ✕		07-Dec-2020

NOTE · · · · · · · · · CHART CHARGE

< Add Note Form Add Text Entry Add Image   Note Details (1/1)

◢ Chief Complaint
  20 Free Text CC

◢ History of Present Illness
  20 Free Text HPI
  Pre-Op Visit
  Text Templates

◢ Review of Systems
  20 Free Text ROS
  Complete-Male
  Text Templates

  Active Problems
  Current Meds
  Allergies
  Past Medical History
  Surgical History

PRE-OP VISIT   ○ Brief ◉ Comprehensive [All Normal] [Previous History]
⌃ Reason for Visit:
  ◉ Preoperative Visit
Procedure Details:
  ☑ Procedure: TKA at cornerston... ☐ Date of Surgery: ___ ☐ Surgeon Name: ___

Indication for Surgery:
  ☑ Indication: knee o...
⌃ Surgical Risk Assessment:
Prior Anesthesia:
  [Y][N] Prior Anesthesia [Y][N] Adverse Reaction, Epidural [Y][N] Adverse Reaction, Spinal
  [Y][N] Adverse Reaction, General

Pertinent Past Medical History:
  ☐ No Pertinent PMHx
  Cardiovascular [Y][N] 2ndary Hypercoagulable State Neurologic
  [Y][N] Angina [Y][N] PE [Y][N] Seizure Disorder
  [Y][N] Arrythmia [Y][N] DVT [Y][N] CVA
  [Y][N] CAD [Y][N] Uses Anticoagulants Pulmonary
  [Y][N] CAD w/Prior MI Metabolic [Y][N] Asthma

View Output « [Sign] ☑ Final [Author ⌄]   Recompile Copy Forward ▾ [Save & Close] [Save] [Close]

```
Assessment and Plan:
Pre-op evaluation (Z01.818)
Plan: Avoid any NSAIDs 7-10 days prior surgery
Patient is MEDICALLY CLEARED TO HAVE a R TKA UNDER GENERAL
ANESTHESIA at Summit Orthopedics.

Primary osteoarthritis of right knee (M17.11)
Impression: Plan correction by R TKA on 12/20/2020 by Dr.
Smith at Summit Orthopedics.
```

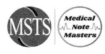

Management of Chronic Diseases

With successful screening strategies, chronic diseases can be identified early and treated. The PCP addresses chronic conditions in multiple stages, from their early beginnings picked up on screening tests, through different treatment strategies, and finally through progress and decline. Although they sometimes seem like "background" issues, active management is required to prevent complications.

Type II Diabetes Mellitus (DM)

There are traditionally two types of diabetes mellitus: Type I and Type II, as shown in the table, but the distinctions are not black-and-white.

Table 6.7: Characteristics of diabetes types

Type I	Type II
Associated with autoimmune antibodies that destroy the pancreatic islet cells that make insulin	No antibodies/not autoimmune
Insulin quantity is low	Insulin is present, but less effective
Diagnosed in youth	Adult-onset, but becoming more frequent in youth
Not associated with obesity	Associated with diet and obesity
Glycemic control can swing widely with eating and insulin administration	Sugar levels less labile, typically hover in high levels
Hypoglycemic episodes occur in patients on insulin	Risk of hypoglycemia very low on PO meds or long-acting insulin
~5% of all cases	~95% of all cases in the US

Type I diabetes is far less common and is usually followed by an endocrinologist as well as a PCP. Type II diabetes, on the other hand, represents the vast majority of diabetes cases and will be the type most commonly seen in a primary care clinic.

Diagnosis of Type II Diabetes Mellitus

The diagnosis of type II diabetes is reasonably straightforward. For most patients, an annual physical exam includes labs like a basic metabolic panel (BMP). Also called a Chem 7, a BMP consists of seven elements that includes blood glucose, and is one of the most commonly ordered blood tests. Sometimes elevated sugars are picked up incidentally on bloodwork or urine ordered for another reason, so

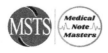

generally if a patient's blood glucose is abnormal on one of these initial tests, then more definitive labs are ordered. The first test may be fasting glucose. Fasting means that this lab is done when the patient has not eaten in several hours, typically overnight, to ensure that a recent meal does not elevate the glucose

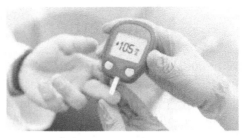

reading. A mildly elevated result is called pre-diabetes (100-125 mg/dL), and a higher result is full diabetes (>126 mg/dL). If at any time glucose is >200, even after a meal, diabetes is quite likely. It may seem odd to diagnose a "pre" disease, but instead think of it in terms of "impaired fasting glucose" or "impaired glucose tolerance" that is likely to progress to diabetes if not managed.

The hemoglobin A1C (or HbA1c) lab test reflects the average blood glucose over 3 months, rather than a single point in time. In the past, it was primarily used for diabetes monitoring, but more recent studies show it is superior to a fasting glucose level for diagnosis as well. The table below shows the ranges for hemoglobin A1C values and the cutoff for normal, pre-diabetes, and a full diagnosis of diabetes.

Table 6.8: Interpretation of A1c results

HbA1c	Interpretation
< 5.8	normal
5.8 - 6.4	Pre-diabetes
> 6.4	Diabetes

HbA1c	Average Blood Glucose
5	90
6	120
7	150
8	180
9	210
10	240

Management and Monitoring of Type II Diabetes

Because A1C levels inform providers about the relative severity, they are used to influence treatment decisions. Well-controlled diabetics with A1Cs below 7 often do well with diet and exercise alone. Diet and exercise are typically recommended first, but medications are soon to follow if sugar control is not achieved. Like other chronic conditions, the physician often starts with common first-line medications, then over time, medications are added and substituted, with compliance, side effects, and efficacy noted. Unfortunately, some people with type II diabetes do

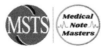

eventually require insulin shots. You do not need to memorize these medications, but again you should be able to recognize the names and spelling and track their use over time in the notes. You may already recognize some from TV advertisements.

Noninsulin Drugs for Type 2 Diabetes Mellitus			
Drug Class (Type)	**Mechanism of Action (How it Works)**	**Drugs Available**	
		Chemical Names	**Brand Names**
Sulfonylureas	Increases insulin secretion by pancreas	glimepiride glipizide	Amaryl* Glucotrol*
		glyburide	Diabeta* Micronase* Glynase*
Biguanides	1) Increases glucose production by the liver 2) Increases uptake of glucose by muscles	metformin	Glucophage*
GLP-1 RAs (glucagon-like peptide-1 receptor agonists)	1) Increases insulin secretion in response to blood glucose level 2) Decreases glucagon secretion by pancreas 3) Delays stomach emptying 4) Increases satiety (i.e. feeling of fullness)	exenatide liraglutide dulaglutide exenatide XR semaglutide lixisenatide	Byetta Victoza Trulicity Bydureon Ozempic Lyxumia
DPP-4 inhibitors (dipeptidyl peptidase-4 inhibitors)	1) Increases insulin secretion in response to blood glucose level 2) Decreases glucagon secretion by pancreas	alogliptin saxagliptin linagliptin sitagliptin	Nesina Onglyza Tradjenta Januvia
TZDs (thiazolidinediones or glitazones)	1) Increases glucose uptake in muscle & fat 2) Decreases glucose production by the liver	pioglitazone rosiglitazone	Actos Avandia
SGLT-2 inhibitors (sodium glucose cotransporter-2 inhibitors)	Increases excretion of glucose in urine by blocking reabsorption in the kidney	canagliflozin empagliflozin dapagliflozin ertugliflozin	Invokana Jardiance Farxiga Steglatro
*also available as a generic preparation			

Table 6.9: Common DM medications. This Photo licensed under CC BY-SA

Complications of Type II Diabetes

We already mentioned the hemoglobin A1C and its utility in monitoring a patient's diabetic control, but there is more to a diabetic clinic visit than just blood sugar numbers. Diabetes can cause widespread damage to small blood vessels, resulting in kidney damage (nephropathy), nerve damage (neuropathy), and eye damage (retinopathy), in addition to raising the risk for general cardiovascular events.

Diabetic nephropathy is kidney damage stemming from long-standing diabetes mellitus ("Neph" refers to the nephron, the functional unit of the kidney). The damage that occurs with diabetes results in larger pores in the filter of the kidney,

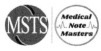

allowing molecules like proteins to leak into the urine. To test for early diabetic nephropathy, a lab for urine microalbumin (a type of protein) is ordered, which is more sensitive than a standard dipstick.

Retinopathy is a disease affecting the small blood vessels within the eye. Diabetic retinopathy is the primary cause of new-onset blindness in adults. Given the risk, diabetic patients require full annual eye exams with an eye specialist to check for early stages of diabetic retinopathy and other eye conditions that are also more common in patients with diabetes – like glaucoma.

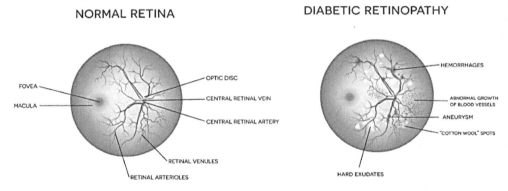

Neuropathy is the loss of sensation or motor function due to damage to a nerve. This often occurs in the feet first, because these are the longest nerves, and the provider will ask about numbness or tingling in the extremities as a sign of neuropathy. Yearly foot exams and monofilament testing evaluate possible diabetic neuropathy. To test the sensory function of the foot, the physician uses a thin plastic filament called a monofilament, places the tip of the filament against a specific region of the foot, and then asks the patient if he or she can feel it. Most EHRs have a specific procedural template to fill out if a provider performs a diabetic foot exam so that this screening test is documented consistently.

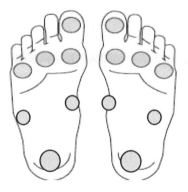

Figure 6.12: Sensory testing sites for the diabetic foot exam

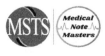

Hypertension

Hypertension, or high blood pressure, is a vascular disease that—like diabetes—predisposes a person to more serious conditions in the future, especially if uncontrolled. Hence, patients with high blood pressure are regularly and routinely seen in the primary care clinic. If normal blood pressure is around 120/70, hypertension, in contrast, is defined as a consistent blood pressure of ≥140/90. Also, like diabetes, hypertension is a widespread systemic disease that can predispose a person to diseases of many organs, as shown in the graphic. Mildly elevated blood pressure is not immediately worrisome. However, if blood pressure is chronically untreated or undertreated, the gradual arterial damage to vital organs (called end-organ damage) can increase the risk of a stroke, heart attack, and chronic kidney disease. For this reason, patients with hypertension require regular monitoring to ensure that the possibility of these complications is minimized.

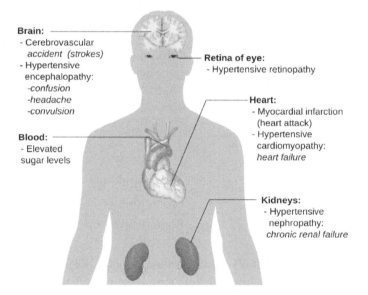

Brain:
- Cerebrovascular
  accident (strokes)
- Hypertensive
  encephalopathy:
  -confusion
  -headache
  -convulsion

Retina of eye:
- Hypertensive retinopathy

Heart:
- Myocardial infarction
  (heart attack)
- Hypertensive
  cardiomyopathy:
  heart failure

Blood:
- Elevated
  sugar levels

Kidneys:
- Hypertensive
  nephropathy:
  chronic renal failure

Figure 6.13: Complications of persistent HTN

Treatment of Hypertension

If a person's average blood pressure meets criteria for hypertension, the patient may be started on a medication to reduce blood pressure. Although the medications may produce the same end-result of BP reduction, they do so via different mechanisms. A patient with persistent hypertension while on one of these medications may

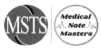

require a second medication from another class—not necessarily just a higher dose of the first medication—to further lower blood pressure. The medications listed here are the most commonly used antihypertensive medications:

- ACE inhibitors like enalapril and lisinopril
- Calcium-channel blockers like amlodipine
- Angiotensin receptor blockers (ARBs) like losartan, olmesartan and irbesartan
- Beta-blockers like atenolol, metoprolol, and carvedilol
- Diuretics like hydrochlorothiazide

Hyperlipidemia

Hyperlipidemia, based on the word roots, is the condition of having high blood lipids. Typically, this refers to abnormally high levels of low-density lipoprotein (LDL) – a risk factor for atherosclerosis (formation of plaque within the arteries) – but it may refer to an elevation of one of the other components of the lipid panel as well. Below are the four major parts of a lipid panel, the range of normal, and the associated condition when a particular component is abnormal.

Table 6.10: Lipid testing ranges

Component	Normal Range	Condition, if outside normal range
Total Cholesterol	< 200	Hypercholesterolemia
LDL	< 100	Hyperlipidemia
HDL	> 40	Dyslipidemia
Triglycerides	< 150	Hypertriglyceridemia

High-density lipoprotein (HDL) is often called "good cholesterol" because higher numbers are desired, and low-density lipoprotein (LDL) is "bad cholesterol" because lower numbers are desired for heart disease prevention. Goal cholesterol levels vary according to the patient's other risk factors for cardiovascular disease (such as DM and HTN), so the interpretation of these numbers varies by patient and should be documented accordingly.

Along with diet, statins are the most commonly used medication to treat hyperlipidemia and related conditions, though others may also be utilized.
1. Statins – Most statins are conveniently named so that the generic name

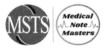

includes the word "statin" within it (e.g., atorvastatin, simvastatin).

2. Fibrates – these medications may be used in conjunction with statins for lipid control, including fenofibrate (Tricor) and gemfibrozil (Lopid).

Changes in a person's lipid profile occur very gradually, so repeat lipid panels are obtained after at least 3 months of initiating statin therapy. However, a follow-up lipid panel may not be repeated for much longer at the provider's discretion.

Hypothyroidism

Hypothyroidism is the condition in which the thyroid gland in the neck is underactive ("hypo" means low). Hypothyroidism often occurs as a result of aging as the thyroid's ability to produce thyroid hormones (T_4 and T_3) diminishes; it is especially common in women over age 60. A simple blood test called the TSH can be used to diagnose hypothyroidism, usually along with the thyroid hormone T4. Thyroid-stimulating hormone (TSH) is a hormone signal to trigger the release of thyroid hormone, so seemingly paradoxically, a low TSH indicates that the thyroid is overactive, and a high TSH indicates that the thyroid is underactive.

Because the thyroid hormones influence metabolic rate, patients with hypothyroidism may report symptoms of fatigue, unexplained weight gain, thinning hair, or depression. Some of screening questions may seem familiar from the ROS section, and positive symptoms would warrant lab testing. Abnormal results may warrant additional tests for an underlying cause, or imaging tests like an ultrasound. Treatment, fortunately, is usually very straightforward with prescription thyroid hormone replacement levothyroxine (Synthroid).

Anxiety and Depression

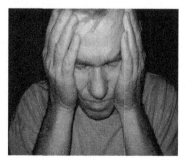

Anxiety and depression often occur together and the treatment overlaps as well, so they are often discussed together. Anxiety is the condition of excess unease or nervousness that is out of proportion to the stimulus, and includes panic, generalized and social anxiety disorders. Depression is a mental state in which patients suffer from a "depressed" (lowered or poor) mood and loss of pleasure in typically enjoyable activities. Up to 20% of Americans experience anxiety, and approximately 7% are diagnosed with

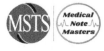

depression, and primary care providers are often the first or only provider a patient sees. Unfortunately, anxiety and depression are often comorbid with other chronic conditions and can make the management of medical disorders more difficult. A patient with uncontrolled depression, for instance, may be less likely to be compliant with diet or medication recommendations, so PCPs mutually address mental and physical health.

The US Preventative Services Task Force has recommended routine screenings for depression so most adult and many adolescent patients receive a screening questionnaire, whether or not the complaint is related to depression. This screening form is called the PHQ-2 and asks how often a patient experiences these symptoms:

1. *Little interest or pleasure in doing things*
2. *Feeling down, depressed, or hopeless*

For patients that have a positive PHQ-2 or have previously been diagnosed with depression, they will be given a more detailed questionnaire known as the PHQ-9. This includes an additional seven questions as below. Each question is scored from 0-3 based how many days the patient experiences symptoms, for a maximum of 27.

3. *Trouble falling asleep, staying asleep, or sleeping too much*
4. *Feeling tired or having little energy*
5. *Poor appetite or overeating*
6. *Feeling bad about yourself-- or that you're a failure, or have let yourself or your family down*
7. *Trouble concentrating on things, such as reading the newspaper or watching TV*
8. *Moving or speaking so slowly that other people could have noticed. Or, being so fidgety or restless that you have been moving around a lot more than usual.*
9. *Thoughts that you would be better off dead or hurting yourself in some way*

Not at all	0
Several days	+1
More than half the days	+2
Nearly every day	+3

Anxiety has a similar screening form known as the GAD-7, meaning it has seven questions about generalized anxiety disorder (GAD). The GAD-7 includes:

1. *Feeling nervous, anxious, or on edge*
2. *Not being able to stop or control worrying*
3. *Worrying too much about different things*
4. *Trouble relaxing*
5. *Being so restless that it is hard to sit still*
6. *Becoming easily annoyed or irritable*
7. *Feeling afraid as if something awful might happen*

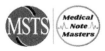

It is graded similarly to the PHQ-9, with 0 being the lowest possible score and 21 being the highest. Most EHRs have templates to input both of these questionnaires, and the score will be classified from mild, moderate or severe. Like all patient evaluations, an interpretation belongs in Results Review or MDM.

Treatment of anxiety and depression includes psychotherapy and/or pharmacologic therapy. Medication management may fall into the hands of the PCP, along with a referral for counseling/therapy, or a psychiatrist can handle both aspects. Referrals to mental health professionals should be documented in the Plan. Several classes of medications are available, as outlined below.

Table 6.11: Common medications for depression and anxiety

Depression	Tricyclics: Amitriptyline (Elavil) Doxepin Imipramine (Tofranil)	Secondary Amines: Desipramine Nortriptyline Protripyline
	NE-dopamine reuptake: Buproprion (Wellbutrin)	Serotonin modulators: Nefazodone (Serzone) Trazodone (Desyrel)
	NE-serotonin modulation: Mirazapine (Remeron)	Monoamine oxidase inhibitors: Phenelzine (Nardil) Moclobemide (Amira)
Anxiety	Buspirone (Buspar) Beta-blockers: Propranolol (Inderal) Atenolol	Benzodiazepines: Alprazolam (Xanax) Clonazepam (Klonopin) Diazepam (Valium) Lorazepam (Ativan)
Anxiety +/- Depression	SSRIs: Citalopram (Celexa) Escitalopram (Lexapro) Sertraline (Zoloft) Fluoxetine (Prozac) Paroxetine (Paxil)	SNRIs: Duloxetine (Cymbalta) Venlafaxine (Effexor)

Many patients will try more than one medication to find something that works, and mentioning prior medications and their effectiveness can be helpful in the HPI or Assessment and Plan. The provider may also provide resources like mental health helplines and ask about any suicidal thoughts. It is vital to document explicitly that the patient does not represent harm to themselves or others, commonly with the phrase "Patient denies suicidal ideation (SI) or homicidal ideation (HI)." If substantial risk is present, the patient may be transferred to an emergency room.

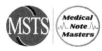

Chronic Low Back Pain

Almost 80% of Americans will experience back pain at some point. Thus, low back pain and the follow-up visits to address and manage it are commonplace. Often, the patient has a prior history of low back problems that should be investigated in the EHR. For worker's compensation cases, extra documentation, including specific work restrictions, is required.

Musculoskeletal causes tend to be more self-limited and are caused by a strain of the muscles in the back or a sprain of the ligaments that bind the vertebrae together. Radicular nerve pains are a bit different. Lumbar radiculopathy and sciatica are similar in that they are caused by compression of a nerve root, but they differ as to where this compression occurs. Compression of a lumbar spinal nerve can result in lumbar radiculopathy – pain that radiates down one of the legs. When it affects the sciatic nerve, a bundle of nerves L4-S3, then it is called sciatica, and pain typically radiates from the buttock to the foot. Recall the straight leg raise from the physical exam section, performed to elicit these types of symptoms.

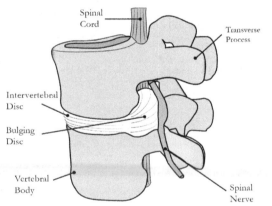

Figure 6.14: Anatomy of a vertebra, disk, and exiting nerve

Treatment of chronic low back pain may involve lifestyle modifications, physical therapy, or the use of muscle relaxants like cyclobenzaprine (Flexeril), NSAIDs, and pain medications. Unfortunately, the use and abuse of controlled substances like opioids have become widespread in the US, and chronic use is discouraged. Most states maintain registries that catalog each person's controlled-substance history, and it is often required that providers consult this registry before prescribing opioids. Some common opioids include:

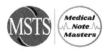

- hydrocodone (found with Tylenol in Vicodin and Norco)
- oxycodone (found with Tylenol in Percocet)
- Oxycontin (extended release form of oxycodone)
- hydromorphone (Dilaudid)
- tramadol (Ultram), which has opioid-like qualities

Many patients who require chronic pain management are referred to chronic pain specialists who often have other treatment options for chronic pain, such as injections and structured opioid-tapering programs.

Common Acute Complaints

Headaches

Nearly everyone has had a headache, but how does the provider know when a garden-variety headache could be something more? Some common headache types will improve on their own, but other types of headaches can be chronic in and of themselves or may be associated with other chronic diagnoses.

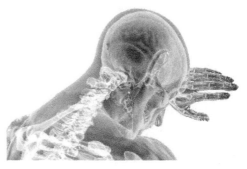

Providers will often first ask about "red flag" symptoms (ones that are associated with dangerous processes):
- Neurologic issues (e.g., confusion, motor weakness, sensory changes)
- Vision changes like double vision or loss of vision
- Fever or infection
- Medical history, including long-term use of anticoagulants (blood thinners), cancer, or weakened immune defenses
- Sudden, severe onset of headache
- History of head trauma or concussion
- Unusually elevated blood pressure

Once the provider determines that dangerous diseases are less likely, he/she can pursue the more common causes in more detail. The provider may ask the patient to keep a "headache diary" to track progress or clarify what is causing or triggering symptoms, such as temporal association with menstruation or eating certain foods.

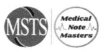

There are three main types of primary headaches.

1. Migraine. Some patients refer to any bad headache as a migraine, but your provider may need to collect more information to determine if the patient meets diagnostic criteria for migraines. Some of these criteria include sensitivity to light (photophobia) or sound (sonophobia), worsening of symptoms with activity, a pulsatile quality to the headache, and nausea/vomiting.

2. Tension Headache. As the name suggests, this type of headache is characterized by a sense of tightness or pressure usually around the head or "hatband."
   Some of the symptoms of tension headaches and migraines are similar, and patients can have both types of headaches at the same time.

3. Cluster Headache. A less common type of headache that recurs in a particular pattern over time (e.g., daily or seasonal pattern). These headaches are classically associated with unilateral facial symptoms like runny nose, eye redness, eye tearing, sweating, or swelling.

Secondary headaches are headaches experienced as part of another primary diagnosis. The patient may not realize that the headache is caused by something else, and the provider may have to do some additional investigation. For instance, headache is a symptom of glaucoma, so the glaucoma is the primary diagnosis.

Headache Treatment

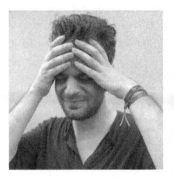

Lifestyle changes may be recommended and can include stress management, improving sleep patterns, modification of caffeine intake, dietary changes, etc. Medications used at the onset of a headache to reduce the symptoms or duration of the headache are called episodic or "abortive" therapies. Common abortive medications include NSAIDs, Excedrin, and triptans. If a patient is using abortive therapies often and is still experiencing headaches, they may be prescribed daily prophylactic medications for migraine prevention such as propranolol, amitriptyline, valproic acid, topiramate, or even Botox.

Upper Respiratory Infections (URIs)

One of the most common reasons a patient presents for evaluation is for an upper respiratory infection, especially during the fall and winter months. Common symptoms of a URI include cough, runny nose, nasal congestion, fatigue and a sore throat. The vast majority of these infections are viral in nature, including variants of the coronavirus, rhinovirus, and others that infect the upper respiratory system diffusely, as opposed to a bacterial infection such as strep that is focused in the oropharynx. URIs are typically spread when an infected person coughs or sneezes,

producing droplets of moisture that contain the virus. Other people then inhale the particles or touch contaminated surfaces, then touch their nose or mouth, allowing the virus to spread. The use of masks on infected persons limits the distance spread of these particles, which can travel a number of feet (as pictured).

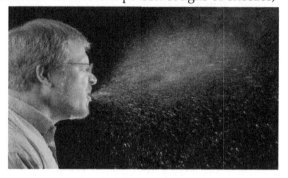

Treatment options

Since most URIs are caused by viruses and effective antiviral therapies are scarce, there is "no cure for the common cold." Thus, a provider will usually recommend symptomatic therapies such as rest and increased fluid intake. Providers may also recommend OTC remedies such as Tylenol for fever or ibuprofen for aches and pains. Decongestants may be used to help decrease nasal congestion, and antitussives may be used for reducing bothersome cough, although most of these therapies are minimally effective. Prescribed inhalers such as albuterol may be helpful for cough even in patients without asthma. If sore throat/pharyngitis is a significant symptom, a strep test may be done. Since strep is a bacterium, if the test is positive, antibiotics will be used. Negative tests are double-checked with a culture, which takes 2-3 days to return.

Antibiotics are not usually recommended for an ordinary URI; however, sometimes a viral URI can linger and reduced defenses may lead to a bacterial infection later on. If a patient has been suffering from URI symptoms for longer than usual (over 2 weeks) or if the patient has immune compromise, the provider may do further tests such as a chest Xray, and antibiotics may be prescribed if there is a high suspicion for bacteria presence. Again, the rationale for ordering or not ordering tests, or prescribing or deferring antibiotics would be documented in the MDM.

Urinary Tract Infections (UTIs)

The vertical ascension of bacteria from the body surface is the main cause of UTIs. Bacteria originating from the bowel or vagina that enters the distal urethra can ascend to the bladder (cystitis), potentially continue up to the kidney (pyelonephritis) or spread systemically (formerly known as urosepsis). UTIs are considerably more frequent in women, as ascending bacteria have a shorter distance to travel to reach the bladder, but prostate enlargement in older men can lead to urinary retention and UTI.

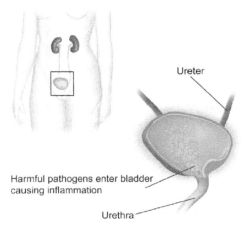

Harmful pathogens enter bladder causing inflammation

Figure 6.15: Cystitis

Bladder infections are the most common type of UTI and may be called cystitis or a lower urinary tract infection. Inflammation of the bladder that occurs with a lower UTI causes a few classic symptoms and signs, including:

- Dysuria—a burning discomfort during urination
- Urinary frequency—increased frequency of urination
- Urinary urgency—the sensation of needing to urinate often
- Hematuria—blood in the urine

If a patient demonstrates a clinical sign of a UTI, then the provider will order a POC urine dipstick or full urinalysis (UA). If the UA is abnormal, the lab may automatically perform a culture to help identify the organism and guide antibiotic therapy, but this requires an extra 24-72 hours. Most cases of cystitis can be treated with a short course of oral antibiotics like Bactrim, Macrobid, or Cipro.

If a lower UTI is left untreated, the infection may progress up a ureter into the kidney(s). This is called pyelonephritis and is colloquially known as a "kidney infection." Clinical symptoms will differ from a bladder infection since the patient often has systemic symptoms like fever, chills, nausea or vomiting along with back pain from the affected kidney. On exam, the provider will assess for costovertebral angle (CVA) tenderness, as this region overlies the kidneys in the mid-back, as opposed to garden-variety musculoskeletal low back pain.

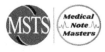

Dermatologic Issues

Dermatologic/skin issues are another one of the most frequent reasons a primary care provider sees patients. Common skin conditions can be handled by the PCP initially, but if problems persist or the issue appears to be more complicated, then the patient may need a referral to a dermatologist or wound-care specialist.

Primary care providers may ask themselves several questions when trying to sort out the type of dermatological issue, such as:

1. Is the problem infectious or non-infectious? Rashes caused by bacteria, fungus, or parasite require treatment specific to the cause, rather than just symptom relief, and precautions to prevent spread are necessary. Providers may ask more detailed questions about possible exposures to seek additional clues.
2. Is the problem allergic or not? Minor allergic reactions to a new detergent or food may result in some hives or localized itching, but more serious allergic reactions can lead to systemic vascular issues, breathing problems, and even death. Due to the possible risk of progressive allergic reactions, the provider may pursue historical elements regarding allergy risk.
3. Is it localized or systemic? Some systemic diseases have skin manifestations, including lupus or diabetes, and can be one of the first diagnostic clues. Similarly, systemic viral infections or systemic immune reactions to medications or foods are treated quite differently than a localized rash.
4. Is it cancerous or benign? Concerning lesions such as moles can be worrisome for cancer or precancerous signs, which require biopsy to differentiate.

If the patient has a puncture, cut, or scrape, tetanus (Tdap) status may be of concern, so proactively look in the EHR for this information.

Physical Exam for Dermatological Issues

Thorough skin exams often involve the provider looking carefully over many parts of the patient's body. If you remain in the room during this portion of a physical exam, be sensitive to the patient's privacy.

For a non-dermatologic complaint, the skin exam might be documented as follows:

"Exposed skin is warm and dry, without lesions."

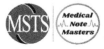

For dermatologic complaints, the description of skin abnormalities can be included in the physical exam where the lesion is located (e.g., a facial rash in the HEENT exam), or it can be included separately in the "skin" or "derm" section. In either case, providers will describe skin lesions both as to how they appear on inspection and how they feel on palpation, because both factor into decision making. Dermatology is very visual, and unless your clinic has photographic equipment, the way visual findings are translated into words in the note is fundamental. Thus, a provider will often dictate the physical exam findings to the scribe with the specific terms desired.

Table 6.12: Common dermatological exam findings

Category	Possible findings
Type	Macular (flat), papular (raised), maculopapular (flat and raised)
Color	Erythematous (red), pale, dark/hyperpigmented, purple, dusky
Shape	Round, linear, irregular, discrete, consistent, variegated
Size	Measure in mm, cm, or approximated
Location	What anatomic areas the lesion overlies, as well as patterns such as clusters or scattered, diffuse
Quantity	Single or multiple
Pattern	Any pattern in location (ex, rash associated with jewelry)
Palpation	Firm, fluctuant (squishy), nodular, warm, dry, or moist
Other	Thickened, scaly, bleeding, purulent (oozing pus), scratch marks

Common Conditions

Rashes: A "rash" is what many patients may call any kind of irritated, red, or itchy skin issue. Unfortunately, at times, the history and physical will not offer a single precise diagnosis, and the assessment may simply be "dermatitis."

Dermatitis: simply means inflammation of the skin. Providers may choose to recommend symptomatic therapies initially. When lacking a diagnosis, carefully document the provider's rationale for starting or postponing treatment.

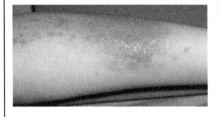

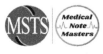

Eczema (i.e. atopic dermatitis): typically causes dry, red, and itchy plaques. It has a familial component and often manifests in childhood. Treatment is centered on anti-inflammatories such as topical corticosteroids or newer, topical or systemic immunomodulatory therapies.	
Psoriasis: a chronic inflammatory disease in which patients most commonly develop thick, itchy plaques over joints like the elbows and knees. Psoriasis is associated with other systemic issues like arthritis, so treatment involves more than just the skin.	
Seborrheic keratosis: Sometimes known as "age spots," these lesions are not cancerous despite sharing a name with actinic keratosis, which are precancerous lesions. Seborrheic keratoses or "SKs" are very common as patients age and typically occur on the face, trunk, and extremities	

Skin Infections: Human skin is usually colonized with several bacterial and fungal organisms, which can cause infections given the right circumstances. Minor trauma or other breakdowns in the skin barrier may introduce a route for bacteria to gain access to deeper skin layers and cause an infection. A reduced immune defense can also make skin infections more likely – especially viral infections of the herpes family that can lead to cold sores and herpes zoster.

Folliculitis: an infection of hair follicles, causing small, round pustules to form around hair follicles. Bacteria from razors and hot tubs are common culprits.	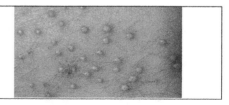

Acne vulgaris: also related to hair follicles, from obstruction and inflammation of the associated oil glands that can also become infected with bacteria.	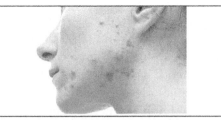
Cellulitis: a diffuse type of skin infection that can begin with reduced skin defense, allowing bacteria to travel beneath the surface level. The skin here is typically firm/indurated and can be bright red or deeper colors.	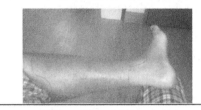
Abscesses and boils: collections of infectious fluid beneath the skin. Because they are fluid-filled, they feel fluctuant or "squishy" on exam. They are treated with a procedure called an Incision and Drainage, in which an incision is made to drain the fluid. Oral antibiotics are not as effective at treating abscesses because there is no blood flow inside a boil.	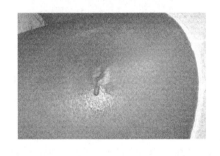
Ulcerations: open sores that develop due to poor circulation, pressure, or injury and more easily become infected. These sores can progress from superficial breakdown of the skin deep into the bone. Foot ulcerations are a concern for diabetic patients due to vascular and nerve damage.	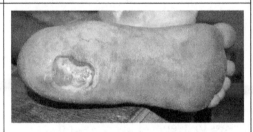
Warts are small, round, raised lesions that typically occur on the hands or feet. When they are located on the bottom of the feet, they are called verruca plantaris. They are caused by the human papillomavirus (HPV) and are more common in patients with weakened immune systems.	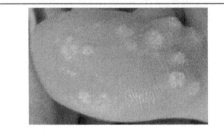

Treatment Options

Many common dermatologic conditions may be handled in a primary care clinic without a dermatology consultation. Common rashes are most often treated with a topical anti-inflammatory cream like hydrocortisone, either prescription or OTC, as well as removing the cause when possible. Fungal infections can also be treated with OTC remedies. Topical or systemic antibiotics are used for infected or possibly infected lesions, and the provider may obtain a culture swab to further identify the bacteria and possible antibiotic resistance. Some providers feel comfortable using cryotherapy to freeze off warts or other lesions, performing a biopsy, or draining an abscess in clinic. Lesions concerning for malignancy might be referred immediately, and the PCP may need to call ahead to expedite the appointment.

Complex Complaints

Most of the visits discussed throughout this chapter may seem relatively straightforward but in reality, this may not be the case. For example, the clinic schedule may list a patient with a chief complaint of cough, which is seemingly simple. After meeting the patient, however, we learn the patient has a long-standing history of smoking, asthma, COPD and coronary artery disease, and suddenly the complexity has significantly increased significantly. All of these relevant histories need to be included, and not only will they increase the complexity, but they will change how a provider will treat the cough. As a scribe, careful documentation of the Assessment and Plan will make it clear why the provider would choose to manage a healthy 19-year-old differently than the patient above.

Another instance of increased complexity is what might initially appear to be an easy medication refill. While these visits can be straightforward, multiple medications mean multiple underlying medical problems and likely multiple prescribers. A patient with hypertension, anxiety, and diabetes may not even remember all of his/her medications and may be experiencing side effects. A helpful scribe will search the EHR and any linked pharmacy databases to assist the physician in populating an accurate medication list.

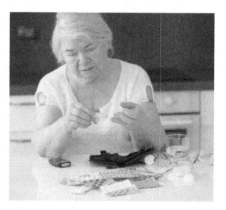

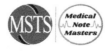

Complete Note – Example 1

You have now read a great deal about medical documentation, but it may be difficult to imagine how all of these elements come together coherently, so review the following examples of complete notes.

CC: Diabetes check

HPI: John Smith is a 47 yo male with a history of type II diabetes and hypertension who presents for a diabetic check. He was last seen in clinic 6 months ago, at which point his A1C was 8.1, and we started him on 500 mg BID metformin. He has been doing well since; no hospitalizations. He checks his blood sugar every morning before breakfast, and it is typically around 105. He denies polydipsia or weight changes. His last eye exam was 1 year ago, and he is due for another, but he denies any visual changes. He denies any lower extremity paresthesias. No new skin ulcers.

ROS: Constitutional: Denies weight changes
Eyes: Denies vision changes
Cardiovascular: Denies chest pain or decreased exercise tolerance.
Neuro: Denies extremity paresthesias, focal weakness
Skin: Denies lesions, rash, pruritis
Endocrine: per HPI

Allergies: Penicillin (rash as a child), peanuts (anaphylaxis)
Medications:
• ASA 325mg QD, Metformin 500 mg BID, Metoprolol 50 mg BID

Past Medical History:
• Diabetes Mellitus, type II (diagnosed 2011)
• Hypertension, chronic
• Pneumonia 2009, resolved

Past Surgical History:
• Appendectomy, 1982
• Right fibula fracture, s/p ORIF, 1985

Family History: Father has hypertension, alive. Mother has type II diabetes, alive. Sister has hypertension but is otherwise healthy. No family history of colon cancer.

Social History: Non-smoker, never has smoked, occasional EtOH. Enjoys tennis for exercise. Works at Wells Fargo.

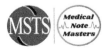

Physical Exam:

Vital Signs: HR: 72, RR: 14, BP: 133/84 Oximetry: 99% RA Weight: 220 lbs (100kg)

GENERAL: Patient is pleasant, well-groomed, well-nourished, no acute distress.

ENT: Normocephalic, atraumatic.

EYES: No conjunctival injection. PERRL, EOMI.

NECK: full ROM, nontender.

RESPIRATORY: Lungs are CTA without wheeze or rhonchi. Good air movement.

CARDIOVASCULAR: Regular rate and rhythm. No murmurs, rubs, or gallops. DP and PT are 2+ and symmetric.

NEUROLOGIC: Awake, alert. Facial movements symmetric. Monofilament exam: Intact sensory function in the feet bilaterally.

PSYCHIATRIC: Normal affect, normal speech.

SKIN: Exposed skin is within normal limits. No ulceration or skin breakdown.

RESULTS:

Basic Metabolic Panel (date):

Sodium	140	[135-145]
Potassium	4.9	[3.5-5.0]
Creatinine	1.0	[0.6-1.2]

Complete Blood Count (date):

WBC	7.8	[4.0-11.0]
Hgb	14.0	[12.0-17.0]
PLTs	370	[140-400]

Mcroalbumin to creatinine ratio:
   40   [30-300]

HgA1C   7.1

Immunizations and Screening exams reviewed in EHR and UTD

Assessment & Plan

1. Type II Diabetes Mellitus – well-controlled with metformin. A1C 7.1, improved from last visit. No evidence of neuropathy or nephropathy today. Continue metformin 500 mg BID. Pt agrees to schedule eye appt. Continue to monitor sugars, encouraged to use a journal. Follow-up in 6 months.
2. Hypertension – well-controlled, continue metoprolol 50 mg BID.
3. Immunizations UTD, plan seasonal flu yearly.
4. Last colonoscopy 2 years ago, GI recommended q5 years.

I, Stephanie Smith, am serving as a scribe to document services personally performed by Michael Parker, MD, based upon my observations and the provider's statements.

I, Michael Parker, MD, attest that I have reviewed and approved the above documentation.

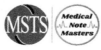

Complete Note – Example 2

Chief Complaint: med check

History of Present Illness: Jamie Jones is a 65 year old F with a history of elevated lipids and PE who presents for a med check. Pt is on chronic anticoagulation medications after a PE in 2019. She is currently taking ASA 81mg PO daily and Xarelto 20mg PO daily. Her hematologist recommended that she stay on oral anticoagulation for her lifetime. She denies any complications on Xarelto, other than easy bruising. She has a PMHx of hyperlipidemia, managed on atorvastatin 10mg PO daily, compliant and w/o side effects. Admits that she experienced myalgias in the past when she was on a higher statin dose, but now resolved. She has a hx of tobacco use and smokes 1 cigarette every 4-5 days.

Information pre-populated from a popup such as an HPI must be changed on that popup to prevent conflicting documentation.

ROS Defaults:

Constitutional ☐ All neg	Cardiovascular ☐ All neg	Reproductive ☐ All neg	Neurological ☐ All neg	Musculoskeletal ☐ All neg
Neg Pos	Neg Pos	Neg Pos	Neg Pos	Neg Pos
○ ○ Chills	○ ○ Chest pain	○ ○ Abnormal Pap	○ ○ Dizziness	○ ○ Back pain
○ ○ Fatigue	○ ○ Claudication	○ ○ Dysmenorrhea	○ ○ Extremity numbness	○ ○ Joint pain
● ○ Fever	○ ○ Edema	○ ○ Dyspareunia	● ○ Extremity weakness	○ ○ Joint swelling
○ ○ Malaise	○ ○ Palpitations	○ ○ Hot flashes	○ ○ Gait disturbance	○ ○ Muscle weakness
○ ○ Night sweats	○ ○ Other:	○ ○ Irregular menses	○ ○ Headache	○ ○ Neck pain
○ ○ Weight gain		○ ○ Vaginal discharge	○ ○ Memory impairment	○ ○ Other:
○ ○ Weight loss		○ ○ Other:	○ ○ Seizures	
○ ○ Other:	Gastrointestinal ☐ All neg		○ ○ Tremors	
	Neg Pos	Integumentary ☐ All neg	○ ○ Other:	Hematologic / Lymphatic ☐ All neg
HEENT ☐ All neg	○ ○ Abdominal pain	Neg Pos		Neg Pos
Neg Pos	● ○ Blood in stools	○ ○ Breast discharge	Psychiatric ☐ All neg	○ ● Easy bruising
○ ○ Ear drainage	○ ○ Change in stools	○ ○ Breast lump	Neg Pos	○ ○ Lymphadenopathy
○ ○ Ear pain	○ ○ Constipation	○ ○ Brittle hair	○ ○ Anxiety	○ ○ Other:
○ ○ Eye discharge	○ ○ Diarrhea	○ ○ Brittle nails	○ ○ Depression	
○ ○ Eye pain	○ ○ Heartburn	○ ○ Hair loss	○ ○ Insomnia	
○ ○ Hearing loss	○ ○ Loss of appetite	○ ○ Hirsutism	○ ○ Other:	Immunologic ☐ All neg
○ ○ Nasal drainage	○ ○ Nausea	○ ○ Hives		○ ○ Contact allergy
○ ○ Sinus pressure	○ ○ Vomiting	○ ○ Pruritus		○ ○ Environmental allergies
○ ○ Sore throat	○ ○ Other:	○ ○ Mole changes	Metabolic / Endocrine ☐ All neg	○ ○ Food allergies
○ ○ Visual changes		○ ○ Rash	Neg Pos	○ ○ Seasonal allergies
○ ○ Other:		○ ○ Skin lesion	○ ○ Cold intolerance	○ ○ Other:
	Genitourinary ☐ All neg	● Other:	○ ○ Heat intolerance	
	Neg Pos	ecchymosis	○ ○ Polydipsia	
Respiratory ☐ All neg	○ ○ Dysuria		○ ○ Polyphagia	
Neg Pos	○ ○ Hematuria		○ ○ Other:	
○ ○ Chronic cough	○ ○ Polyuria (Genitourinary)			
● ○ Cough	○ ○ Urinary frequency			
○ ○ Known TB exposure	○ ○ Urinary incontinence			
○ ○ Shortness of breath	○ ○ Urinary retention			
○ ○ Wheezing	○ ○ Other:			
○ ○ Other:				

● All others negative

Save & Close   Cancel

Allergies: Simvastatin → myalgias at high dose
Medications: atorvastatin 10 mg po qd
      Xarelto 20 mg po qd
      ASA 81 mg po qd

Past Medical History:

Tobacco Dependence	h/o pulmonary embolism	Hyperlipidemia
Cataract NEC	Atherosclerosis L carotid	h/o colonic polyp

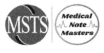

Past Surgical History: hiatal hernia repair and fundoplication
Tonsillectomy
ACL, MCL
1. Left total knee arthroplasty.   12/05/2018

Family History:
Mother breast cancer, advanced age. Father COPD d/t smoking.

Social History:
1-2 cigarettes q4-5 days x 15 years. Lives independently with husband, retired.

Exam:

Date	Time	Ht (in)	Wt (lb)	BMI	BP	Position	Pulse	Resp	Temp (F)	Pulse Ox Rest
12/02/2020	7:55 AM	64.50	210.60	35.59	136/86		69	16	94.60	95

Constitutional: well-developed, NAD, obese
HEENT: PERRL. Oropharynx unremarkable.
Respiratory: CTA bilaterally. No increased WOB.
Cardiovascular: regular rate and rhythm. Cap refill wnl x 4 extremities.
Neurologic: alert, oriented, memory intact
Psychiatric: appropriate mood and affect.
Skin: no petechiae, no visible ecchymosis
Musculoskeletal: no c/c/e, calves nontender

Assessment and Plan:

Assessments			
My Plan	1.	Assessment	Hyperlipidemia, unspecified hyperlipidemia type (E78.5), chronic.
A/P Details		Impression	Labs on 11/25/2020 showed total cholesterol of 170, HDL of 80, an LDL of 82, and triglycerides at 86.
Labs		Patient Plan	LDL goal is <70.
Diagnostics			Increase atorvastatin from 10mg PO daily to 20mg PO daily. If pt experiences myalgias, will decrease dose back to
Referrals			10mg.
Office Procedures			Labs reviewed today.
Review/Cosign Orders	2.	Assessment	Long term (current) use of anticoagulants (Z79.01), chronic.
View Immunizations		Patient Plan	Continue Xarelto 20mg PO daily and ASA 81mg PO daily.
Office Diagnostics			
Physical Therapy Orders	3.	Assessment	Tobacco dependence (F17.200), Active.
Health Promotion Plan		Impression	Pt smokes 1 cigarette every 4-5 days.
Community Resources		Patient Plan	Cessation discussed.
	4.	Assessment	BMI 35.0-35.9, adult (Z68.35), Active.
		Patient Plan	Recommended a 20-lb weight loss.
			Healthy diet and exercise discussed.

I, James Jones, served as a scribe to document services performed by Jerry Orobach, MD, based upon my observations and the provider's statements.

I, Michael Parker, MD, attest that I have reviewed and approved the documentation entered by the aforementioned scribe prior to note finalization and signature.

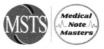

End of Chapter Quiz

1. Bone density testing is primarily done in _____women.
    a. Adult
    b. Post-menopausal
    c. Teenage
    d. Elderly

2. Osteoporosis can be treated with which of the following items?
    a. Calcium
    b. Vitamin D
    c. Alendronate
    d. All of the above

3. Monofilament testing assesses for early signs of _____, a condition associated with type II diabetes mellitus.
    a. Hypertension
    b. Nephropathy
    c. Neuropathy
    d. Retinopathy

4. Diabetic nephropathy is assessed via which of these tests?
    a. Monofilament testing
    b. Hemoglobin A1c
    c. Lipid panel
    d. Urine microalbumin

5. True or False: Hypertension is defined as a blood pressure of greater than 140/90 on a single measurement.
    a. True
    b. False

6. Which medication below is NOT used to treat type II diabetes?
    a. Atorvastatin
    b. Glimepiride
    c. Glipizide
    d. Metformin

7. A "kidney infection" is more technically known as what?
    a. Peptic ulcer disease
    b. Nephrosis
    c. Nephrolithiasis
    d. Pyelonephritis

8. Which medication is not an opioid?
    a. Dilaudid
    b. Morphine
    c. Hydrocodone
    d. Hydrochlorothiazide

9. Which questionnaires are used to gauge a patient's likelihood of having depression?
    a. GAD-7; PHQ-2
    b. TSH; A1c
    c. PHQ-9, GAD-7
    d. PHQ-2; PHQ-9

10. Which diagnostic study is NOT usually part of the normal screening recommendations for a 70-year-old patient?
    a. DEXA scan
    b. PSA
    c. Colonoscopy
    d. Mammogram

11. True or False: A low TSH level is indicative of hypothyroidism.
    a. True
    b. False

Answers: 1. B 2. D 3. C 4. D 5. B 6. A 7. D 8. D 9. D 10. B 11. B

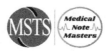

6B. The Emergency Department

Called either the emergency department (ED) or the emergency room (ER), the ED sees a wide variety of patients, and the environment can be drastically different at

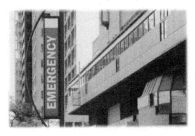

different times of day and in different locations. Most ERs are within or attached to a hospital so that ill patients have the hospital's full resources available next door, but more recently, "stand-alone" ERs and urgent cares have arisen as well. Many EDs have upwards of twenty beds that can be in use at any time, some for general use and others with specialized equipment. An ED typically has a few large trauma bays reserved to accommodate required staff and equipment. There may also be rooms reserved for dental complaints, eye complaints, ob/gyn complaints, and psychiatric complaints because of the specialized equipment required for each of these cases. A large track board screen is often in a central location, or on each computer's home screen, so that the status of every room in the ED can be seen in a single view.

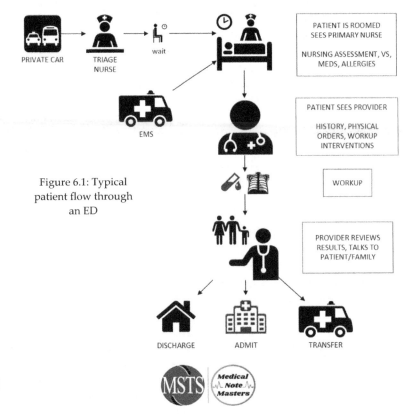

Figure 6.1: Typical patient flow through an ED

Emergency Department Personnel

The ED has a lot of moving parts and requires a variety of specialized staff to work together smoothly. Larger EDs often color-code scrubs, to make it easier to recognize each person's role quickly visually.

Physicians

This is a group of physicians with MD or DO credentials, preferably board-certified in emergency medicine, who provide services in the ER. Other specialists like surgeons may be intermittently present as well. ED physicians manage multiple patients concurrently, and the scribe must track their multitasking.

Midlevel Provider

"Midlevels" such as nurse practitioners (NP) or physician assistants (PA-C) are licensed to diagnose and treat patients under the supervision of a physician.

Triage Nurse

Triage nurses see incoming patients and perform a brief assessment to determine how urgently medical attention is needed. Then, based on priority, the patient may be roomed in the ED or placed back in the waiting room.

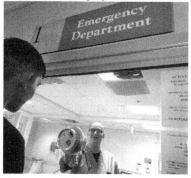

ED Nurse (RN, LPN, APRN)

After rooming, this nurse is responsible for caring for the patient. He or she will perform an initial evaluation of the patient, including a review of the patient's current medications and allergies, place the patient on cardiac or pulse oximetry monitors as needed, and then administer medications per protocol and later as ordered by the physician. One nurse may have up to 4-5 patients at a time, depending on local or union policy.

Charge Nurse

The head nurse in the ED or hospital who assigns tasks to other nurses and deals with patient admissions and transfers. The charge nurse ensures smooth patient flow in the ED but does not routinely directly assist with patient care.

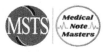

Nursing Supervisor

Also known as "nursing supe," this individual oversees overall hospital census and nurse staffing, and may oversee ancillary staff as well.

Health Unit Coordinator (HUC) or Unit Secretary

The HUC often sits in a central area to assist in multiple administrative functions like paging physicians, arranging transportation, obtaining medical records, and coordinating orders with lab and radiology.

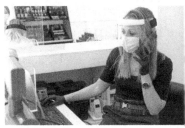

ED Tech

ED technicians ("techs") perform various tasks such as assisting patients, splint placement, laceration set-up, vital sign checks, and many other duties within the ED. Their responsibilities vary greatly in different locations.

Radiology Tech

The radiology technicians are staff members that perform imaging studies such as x-rays, CT scans, and ultrasounds. They may assist with transferring a patient room to the radiology area as well.

Laboratory Tech

The laboratory technician is a staff member that collects samples such as blood and urine and takes them to the lab for analysis.

Emergency Medical Services (EMS)

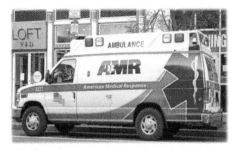

EMS staff transport patients in the ambulance and are trained in emergency response, including some medical procedures. EMTs/medics also sometimes perform tasks in the ED and can be employees of the hospital. There are varying levels of EMS training, ranging from technicians to full paramedics.

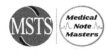

The Emergency Department Process

1.Mode of Arrival

Patients arrive at the ED via a variety of mechanisms: walk-in, private vehicle, non-emergent medical transport, EMS, or even just wheeled over from an adjacent clinic. Mode of arrival is typically documented in the note because it can be an indicator of how emergent the visit will be. When presenting per EMS, the crew will sign off to the receiving nurse or physician, and leave a "run sheet" or similar documentation of their time with the patient. The run sheet can contain valuable information such as blood sugar measurements, VS, and medications administered that must be captured in the note.

2. Triage

Patients presenting to the front door will first be evaluated in triage, where they are assessed briefly to determine the urgency of their condition. Triage is the entry point to the main ED for patients arriving by car or on foot. If the patient presents via ambulance, EMS has already triaged the patient, so they bypass triage and often enter via a separate entrance.

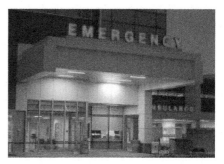

EMTALA is a federal law that requires EDs to evaluate and stabilize anyone who presents, regardless of their ability to pay. This usually means that no matter the reason, every person coming through the front door will go through triage for initial assessment and have an opportunity to see a provider (after a wait).

3. ED Room Placement

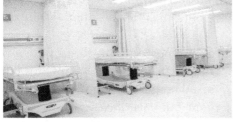

When a patient is up next to be seen, he or she is escorted to a particular room or bay number. Depending on the complaint, the patient may be asked to provide a urine sample, change into a gown, be connected to monitors, or other basic preparation.

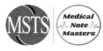

4. Initial Nursing Evaluation

After rooming, the primary nurse takes over and performs a more in-depth evaluation of the patient. He/she documents findings in the EHR but there is a delay, so the physician may check the EHR or ask the nurse personally what was found. Nurses may initiate some workup, like an EKG or blood sugar, based on protocol.

5. Initial Physician History and Physical Exam

At this point, or even earlier, the provider will perform the initial patient assessment. Upon entering the room, things may move very quickly, so stay on your toes! Depending on your facility, you may take short-hand notes on a clipboard or document directly into the EHR with a laptop or mobile computing station.

After the initial assessment, the provider will take a few minutes to explain the upcoming workup plan to the patient, such as labs or imaging to be done. This explanation often includes elements of the Clinical Decision Making that the scribe should capture. After stepping out of the room, the provider may dictate further details to the scribe, such as physical exam abnormalities.

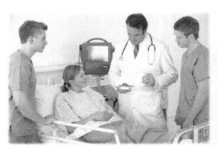

6. The Workup

The physician now enters orders for the planned workup, which commonly includes blood tests and radiology studies. Once the orders are in, a variety of ED personnel will work with the patient to accomplish these tasks and then await results. This creates a "pause" that can be relatively long, particularly if services are backed up, so the physician will move on to see the next patient or wrap up current patients. The MDM may be in two parts, with an "Initial Impression" that reflects the rationale before workup, and a second portion for the rationale after workup.

Nearly everything in the workup portion will be documented in the Results Review or Clinical Course – even if the physician did not personally perform it. For example, a nebulizer administered by respiratory therapy might go unnoticed by the scribe following a physician from room to room, but nevertheless, ALL ordered interventions require documentation. Fortunately, the EHR enables you to see everything that has been ordered in the workup, so you should not miss anything.

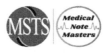

6.5 Possible Sign-out

ED physicians work in shifts, so one physician may begin seeing a patient but then sign out continuing care to the next shift. This occurs most often during the "workup" phase, while awaiting results, but can occur at other times as well. Sign-out is a notoriously risky practice, since it is difficult to adequately convey to the oncoming shift precisely what has happened so far, and physicians may have substantially different approaches. In these cases, careful documentation is crucial as always, and additional notation is required to clarify that physician A is signing out to physician B, workup C is pending, and the plan is X if the workup is normal and Y if the workup is not. Many physicians will evaluate the patient anew, to ensure that nothing is missed, so physician B's note may contain his or her own review of the HPI and exam, or simply the A&P.

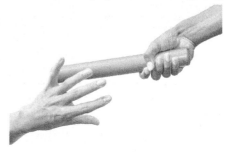

7. Procedures

Some patients require a procedure during their visit—such as lacerations, dislocations, fracture alignment, nosebleed packing, or more serious interventions like cardiac resuscitation. Procedures performed in the ED by the ED physician are documented in the physician note in a specific format. Because procedures involve additional patient risk and physician work, proper documentation is required to clarify patient safety measures and coding items. (Billing and reimbursement are discussed further in Chapter 7.)

Most EHRs will have a template for entering procedures, with required fields marked so you do not accidentally omit them. Procedures performed outside the ED, or by another provider physically in the ED (like a plastic surgeon repairing a wound), are simply documented as an event in the ED Course.

In the following example, a patient undergoes a shoulder relocation under conscious sedation, so Doctor A enters the procedure note for sedation, and Doctor B enters the procedure note for the shoulder relocation. Sedation is considered a form of anesthesia, and because it is riskier than most procedures, this would be a more complicated procedure note.

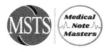

Procedure Note: Conscious Sedation
Indication: R shoulder dislocation
Universal protocol observed with time-out, correct site, and patient confirmed.
Performed by: sedation [self], shoulder reduction Dr. B
Consent: written informed consent obtained from patient and placed on chart
ASA class: [I-IV]
Mallampati Score: [1-4]
Last po intake: *** hours ago
Medications administered: ***
Procedure: Monitoring: Continuous monitoring of HR, RR, pulse oximetry and ETCO2. Supplemental oxygen administered prior to and during procedure via nasal cannula. Resuscitation equipment at the bedside during sedation.
Complications: No desaturations occurred. The patient recovered from the sedation without complication or incident. Patient returned to pre-sedation level of awareness. The monitoring was discontinued at this time.
Start time: ***
End time: ***
Patient tolerated procedure well with good pain control.

8. Re-evaluations

Patients are reevaluated on a semi-routine basis by the physician and nursing staff throughout the visit. The patient's condition is not "on pause" while awaiting workup results – neurologic symptoms wax and wane, pain may worsen, blood pressures can drop, heart rates fluctuate, etc. Without careful documentation of these changes in the Clinical Course, it might appear to someone reading the note that the "pause" was completely uneventful.

As labs and other results roll in, the patient may need re-examined, or additional orders may need to be placed. Since the ED physician can be juggling ten patients in different stages of workup, it is usually helpful if the scribe alerts the physician when new results appear. When interventions such as medications or therapies are given, the physician may need to re-examine the patient to determine if the intervention was effective. A common example would be a repeat pulmonary exam

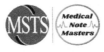

after a nebulizer treatment. A complete note includes documentation of these updates with the time they occurred (called a timestamp) recorded in the ED course.

In a busy shift, the scribe may not always be able to keep up with the physician and have time to type up the note in real-time. In these instances, the physician may update you verbally what has happened while you are at a computer typing up a different patient.

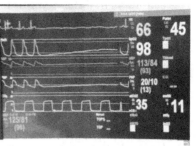

Figure 6.2: Cardiac monitoring This Photo is licensed under CC BY-SA

9. Consultations

Patients present to the ED with an unpredictable, wide variety of issues, so the ED physician may need to consult with a specialist for assistance. Frequent specialist consultations occur with surgeons, cardiologists, gastroenterologists, and mental health professionals. The consult may be over-the-phone, over telemedicine conferencing, or in-person if the consultant is physically available to see the patient. ED physicians may also consult with other services like detoxification facilities and poison control. The health unit coordinator (HUC) pages on-call specialists for the ED provider and may track call-back times. Hearing the physician ask the HUC to "page ortho" is your clue that a consult is about to occur. The scribe needs to note the name of the consultant(s) and the recommendations provided, either by observing the consult or having the ED physician dictate the summary to you later.

10. Assessment and Plan (A&P – see Chapter 5)

Finally, the visit culminates in the assessment and plan. The physician evaluates all of the information gathered, makes a diagnosis, determines the most appropriate

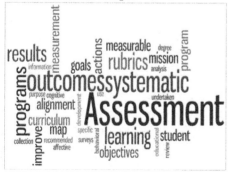

plan, and discusses it with the patient. For complex patients, the thought process that formulated the A&P is written out in the Medical Decision-Making (MDM) paragraph. The MDM and A&P contain the most valuable medical input, and as a scribe, you can learn a great deal from listening carefully to how this is explained to the patient or further explained to you.

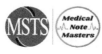

11. Disposition

The planned final destination of the patient is called the "disposition" or "dispo." The physician most often enters the disposition as an order, which triggers a change on the ED track board. In EHR terms, the choices are as below:

- Admission – to the current inpatient facility
- Discharge – to the patient's home, assisted care, nursing home, mental health or chemical dependency facilities, jail, or the morgue
- Transfer – transported to a parallel or higher level of care

Discharge home and admission are the most common dispositions. Prior to discharge, the ED physician will explain the A&P to the patient, so the scribe can denote much of the MDM and A&P in the note by translating this explanation into medical terms. Admissions are inherently more complex patients, so these notes will incorporate the Plan explained to the patient but should also have a clear MDM explaining why admission is needed. Your documentation needs to be promptly entered into the EHR so that the admission team has the information readily available, and should include the name of the admitting doctor.

Patients may also be transferred to a different hospital for more specialized care if necessary, and this process is notoriously risky, so documentation should be prompt and thorough and at the very least include the following:

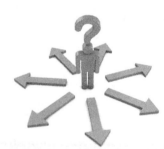

- Who accepted the patient at the other facility.
- What the diagnosis/pressing medical issue is.
- Where exactly the patient is going.
- The timeline of transfer arrangements.
- How the patient is getting there.
- Why the transfer is needed (e.g., your hospital lacks the required service).

The physician and the patient may not always agree as to disposition. Most disagreements occur when the patient declines a physician's recommendation for admission, and insists upon going home instead. The provider will emphasize the risk of going home and determine if the patient is of sound mind to make the decision. If a mentally competent patient still decides to leave, staff will ask the patient to sign a form acknowledging that risks/benefits have been discussed and he/she still chooses to leave against medical advice (AMA). A sample AMA

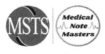

documentation phrase is below, and like procedure consent, there are legal implications. Some patients simply leave the ER without warning, and a disposition of "eloped" or "left without being seen (LWBS)" may be entered.

> The patient chooses to leave AMA. This patient appears to be of sound mind and competent to refuse medical care. The patient is not psychotic, delusional, suicidal, homicidal or hallucinating. The patient is clinically sober and does not appear to be under the influence of any illicit drugs. The patient was strongly encouraged to stay and has been advised of the risks of leaving AMA which include, but are not limited to: death, permanent disability, loss of function, delay in diagnosis. The patient understands that he/she may return at any time for further care. The patient ***did/did not*** sign AMA paperwork.

Alternatively, some patients cannot be allowed to leave due to intoxication, confusion, or psychiatric conditions that would pose a safety danger outside of medical supervision. For example, if a distraught suicidal patient is escorted by police to the ER, the physician will sign a medical hold, sometimes called a 72-hour hold, to keep the patient from leaving until a more formal psychiatric evaluation can occur. Likewise, an intoxicated patient may be placed on a hold until sobriety occurs or a responsible adult can care for the patient at home. To prevent a patient from escaping, restraints such as medications, straps, security presence or a locked room may be required. Since these situations involve involuntarily removing a 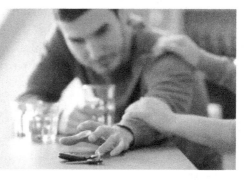 patient's' freedoms, careful documentation is required to demonstrate why restraints were required and that patient safety was paramount.

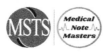

Common Emergency Medicine Conditions

The emergency room is open 24 hours a day, 7 days a week, 52 weeks a year. ER physicians are jacks of all trades, tasked with treating patients with a wide variety of complaints. Many patients cannot – and need not – be definitively managed in a single ER visit, so the physician must decide whether the patient's complaint represents 1) something dangerous that requires admission/transfer, or 2) a condition that can safely be treated as an outpatient with appropriate follow-up.

An emergency physician does not necessarily first try to diagnose the exact cause of a patient's symptoms (and often they cannot due to time and resource constraints), but at the minimum, **rule out** something potentially dangerous. This logic is inherent in the fact that the patient presented to the EMERGENCY room, so the provider must assume first that something dangerous is afoot. For example, for a chief complaint of headache, the physician might first think of intracranial bleeding. This is not the most likely reason by far, but it is among the reasons most likely to be immediately dangerous, so these dangerous diagnoses are ruled out first with a combination of clinical logic and workup. Thus, knowing the basic features of the "rule out" process helps the scribe understand the reasons physicians ask the questions they do, why they examine particular things, why certain tests are ordered, and finally, why the physician arrives at a conclusion and plan. The MDM reflects this process as well, explaining why the physician thought the cause was NOT dangerous diagnosis X, Y or Z. Some physicians make this process seem natural and straightforward, but the process takes skill and years to understand. Working as a scribe, watching this process over and over, gives you a significant head start for your own future clinical logic.

You may wonder how much medical knowledge you really need to know to be a scribe, and we believe that having a basic foundation of medical concepts helps form a coherent note. Also, most scribes are interested in healthcare fields, so learning some medicine now may be valuable later. If you cannot absorb all of this before your first day of work, that is understandable—simply come back and review the materials again. A great note demonstrates flow of thought and tells a story. That is, the note is arranged in such a way that the clinical logic is evident to someone else reading it. You may not be able to accomplish this on day one, but over time, your goal is to write the note the same way the physician would have.

Let's begin with some common ED chief complaints.

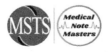

Chest Pain and Cardiac Disease

Chest pain (CP) is one of the most common complaints for patients presenting to the emergency department, and you will be writing many CP notes. The pain might be from any number of causes, such as a myocardial infarction, musculoskeletal strain, or just anxiety. Myocardial infarctions (MIs) and pulmonary embolisms (PEs), however, are amongst the two most potentially fatal causes of chest pain, so we will detail the pathophysiology, signs, symptoms, and tests that differentiate between these two need-to-know rule-out conditions.

Myocardial Infarction (MI)

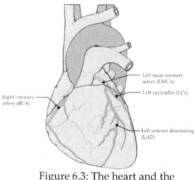

A "heart attack" occurs when an artery supplying the heart muscle (coronary artery) is clogged or too narrowed to provide sufficient blood flow. This causes impaired oxygen delivery to the heart muscles, reducing their ability to contract and leading over time to cellular death. Any condition that causes vascular damage predisposes a person to an MI, including age, diabetes, smoking, HTN, and hyperlipidemia. Once an artery is narrowed by

Figure 6.3: The heart and the coronary arteries

greater than 70%, a patient may experience chest pain with exercise that subsides with rest (angina). If the stenosis is more severe (> 90%), blood flow may be so limited that a patient experiences chest pain even at rest (unstable angina).

The workup for patients with chest pain will begin with an electrocardiogram, or EKG/ECG. An EKG evaluates the electrical conduction of the heart and detects cardiac damage because those areas do not conduct electricity normally. The most recognizable alteration in conduction are changes in the S and T waves becoming elevated or depressed. Without knowing how an EKG works, you will still be able to see this difference in the following two EKG snippets.

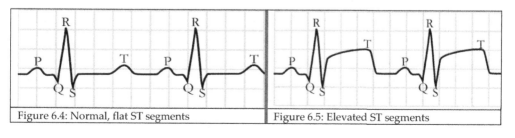

| Figure 6.4: Normal, flat ST segments | Figure 6.5: Elevated ST segments |

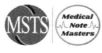

In cases where ST-elevation is seen clearly, it is called an ST-elevation myocardial infarction (STEMI) and most hospitals have a "STEMI protocol" or "Code STEMI" that mobilizes multiple teams in the hospital for STAT response. As a scribe, you are also on high alert because these protocols require very specific documentation, sometimes on paper or in a specific EHR form.

In addition to one or more EKGs, providers will order a lab test looking for indicators of cardiac cell death in the bloodstream called troponin. When cardiac muscle cells die, they release troponin into the blood; however, it takes hours to be detectable. Because of this delay, a patient presenting shortly after the onset of chest pain will need serial troponin measurements over time. If the EKG or the troponin is abnormal, a patient may need emergent cardiac intervention to open or bypass the blocked artery. Other treatments include oxygen, nitroglycerin, aspirin or stronger anti-clotting medications, and medications to lower HR.

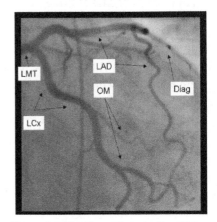

Even if the workup is negative, some patients with multiple risk factors will still be admitted to the hospital for further evaluation because their risk is too high to be safely sent home.

Figure 6.6: Cardiac catheterization. This Photo is licensed under CC BY-SA

Understanding this process will help summarize relevant information from prior ED visits and hospital admissions. For example, if you are seeing a patient with left-sided chest pain, and you see that he/she was admitted to the ED two days ago for this same pain, you should now have the knowledge to write something like this:

> *"John Doe is a 53-year-old male with a history of HTN and hyperlipidemia who presents with recurrent left anterior chest pain. He was admitted with similar chest pain two days ago and had a negative workup including EKG, serial troponins, chest x-ray, and stress echo..."*

Understanding the classic presentation for an MI will be beneficial to your work. Similarly, specifying pertinent negatives such as "patient denies exertional symptoms, no diaphoresis... no history of smoking, HTN, DM, high cholesterol, or family history" helps outline the clinical logic deeming the patient to be lower risk.

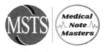

Pulmonary Embolism (PE)

An embolus is something that starts in one place but later breaks away and moves elsewhere. A PE is caused by the formation of a thrombus/blood clot that moves from its original site and becomes lodged in a lung blood vessel. When the clot lodges in the lung tissue, symptoms can begin relatively suddenly.

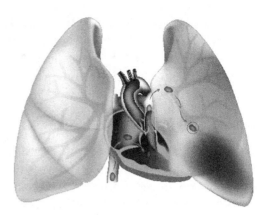

To have a PE, one must first form the blood clot. Patients are predisposed to

Figure 6.7: PE schematic.

forming thrombi by immobility, surgery, smoking, cancer, genetic conditions and other risk factors. Most often, the culprit clot starts in a deep lower leg vein because the flow is more stagnant, and this is called a deep vein thrombosis (DVT). The lower leg may have telltale signs of tenderness and swelling on exam, so the extremity exam needs to be documented on chest pain patients even though it may seem unrelated.

Once the thrombus has formed, it may stay put, or it may dislodge and travel through the venous system all the way back to the heart. From there, it is pumped out to the pulmonary circulation. The clot now encounters increasingly narrower blood vessels, so it becomes lodged, causing signs and symptoms of PE:

1. The patient begins feeling symptoms of pain and shortness of breath, the severity of which can vary widely based on the size of the clot and the patient's underlying pulmonary health.
2. Pain location varies as well, depending on where the clot lodged. It is often described as pleuritic, meaning that it is worse with breathing.
3. Heart rate increases, since the heart now pumps against a clogged vessel. Heart strain and hypoxia may lead to EKG changes.
4. Because blood from the heart is no longer reaching all of the lung regions for gas exchange, the patient may become hypoxic (low oxygen).
5. Pulmonary tissue death will contribute to hypoxia as the lung tissue becomes incapable of participating in respiration. Death and degradation of lung tissue may lead to a very concerning sign of a PE—hemoptysis (coughing up blood).

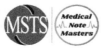

Along with routine chest pain testing like lab tests, EKG, and chest Xray, the physician may consider a blood test called a d-dimer. Elevated levels of d-dimer can indicate a blood clot is lurking somewhere, but it is not specific. A lower extremity ultrasound to look for DVT may also be ordered. If suspicion remains high, a chest CT angiogram (CTA, "angio" refers to blood vessels) more directly tests for PE.

Chest Pain Differential

While we focused on coronary disease and PE, these are only two of many causes of chest pain. Other dangerous causes include diseases of the aorta and heart valves or pulmonary diseases like pneumonia or a collapsed lung. Most patients will have a more benign cause, such as cartilage inflammation (called costochondritis), anxiety, or GERD. Again, the MDM will perhaps cover a number of the other possible diagnoses and the rationale of arriving at the diagnosis chosen. For instance, documenting that the chest pain is sharp, worse with coughing, and constant for 2 weeks, and reproduced with palpation over the rib cartilage covers the positive findings. Further documenting that the physician considered a PE but believes it was NOT a PE due to the duration, associated symptoms, exam findings and workup results solidifies the "rule-out" rationale. We cannot cover everything here, but this will get you off to a start regarding the thought process of chest pain documentation.

Table 6.1: OPQRST Comparison of two dangerous causes of chest pain

	Myocardial Infarction	Pulmonary Embolism
Onset	Gradual or sudden	Sudden
Provoking factors	Exertion	Inspiration, exertion
Palliating factors	Rest, nitroglycerin	Possibly rest
Quality	Pressure	Sharp
Radiation	Left jaw, neck, arm	Usually none
Severity	Varies	Varies
Timing	Crescendo, stuttering	Worst at onset, then constant
Associated signs/sx	Diaphoresis, nausea	Hemoptysis, tachypnea, tachycardia

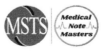

Abdominal Pain

The abdominal cavity is a conglomeration of organs, predominantly parts of the gastrointestinal system. For ED physicians, abdominal pain can be difficult to diagnose in a single visit definitively, so the rule-out methodology is used. We will overview the essential "rule-out" conditions that commonly locate to a particular location in the abdomen and the features that differentiate amongst them.

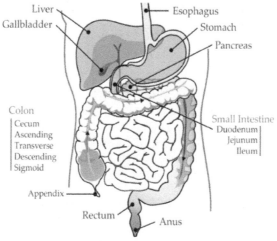

Figure 6.8: Abdominal organs

Generalized pain

Patients often have some difficulty localizing abdominal pain and may report pain "all over." In some ways this is reassuring, because it indicates that no one single organ is severely affected, but in patients presenting in medical distress, it is more concerning because it indicates a widespread problem.

Abdominal fluids

Fluids within the abdominal cavity can flow from area to area, leading to non-localized symptoms. Some fluid is healthy for lubrication of the organs, but abnormal fluids can be worrisome. Internal bleeding leads to blood in the abdominal cavity, as could be the case with ectopic pregnancies, trauma, or ruptured vessels. Patients with liver disease develop excess abdominal fluid called ascites, which can be problematic in itself but can also get infected. Fluids can be detected on CT scan or ultrasound in radiology, but that takes time, so the ED physician may choose to do an ultrasound at the bedside to check for abnormal fluids urgently.

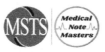

Bowel Obstruction

In a bowel obstruction, solid, liquid, or gaseous contents cannot pass through an obstructed point, and complications will occur from the blockage. As the intestine swells, intestinal contents begin backing up, and the abdomen becomes distended. A bowel obstruction usually causes nausea and cramps with the intake of even small amounts of food. In later stages, bowel obstructions cause generalized pain, nausea, and "tinkling" bowel sounds, and can be diagnosed by Xray or CT scan.

The Left Lower Quadrant (LLQ)

The primary organ residing within the LLQ is the colon (i.e. the large intestine or bowel), along with some components of the genitourinary system. Note that kidney stones and ovarian pathologies (discussed later) could also cause pain in the lower abdominal quadrants, but their presentations are quite different.

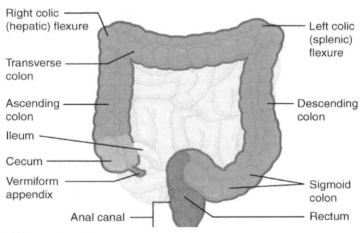

Figure 6.9: The colon. This Photo licensed under CC BY

Colitis

Colitis is inflammation of the colon, and while inflammation is not always from infection, infectious colitis is the most frequently encountered type. Bacteria abound in the colon, but when they are able to invade the wall of the colon, inflammation and pain result. Patients with colitis will often have a fever, elevated WBC, and episodes of diarrhea (sometimes with blood or mucus). An abdominal CT will reveal intestinal wall thickening from the inflammation. With widespread antibiotic use, particularly in healthcare facilities, a bacterium called *C. diff* is becoming more prevalent and more challenging to treat. A stool sample may be obtained to test for *C. diff* or other unusual bacteria. Patients with colitis will typically be treated with oral antibiotics metronidazole (Flagyl) and ciprofloxacin (Cipro).

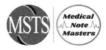

Diverticulitis

Diverticulitis is similar to colitis, but it occurs in small pouches or protrusions in the colon called diverticula (singular diverticulum). These pockets may trap fecal matter, where bacteria can hide out and multiply rather than being passed with bowel movements. Proliferation in this pocket eventually starts inflaming the colon wall in this localized region and can form an abscess. Because the inflammation is more localized than colitis, patients may present with milder symptoms and may not have a fever or elevated WBC. An abdominal CT makes the diagnosis of diverticulitis, and stool samples are unlikely to aid in the diagnosis. Diverticulitis is treated with similar antibiotics to colitis along with bowel rest (liquid diet).

Constipation

Constipation is one of the most frequent causes of LLQ discomfort, especially in children and the elderly, and is basically the excess accumulation of stool within the colon. When hard dry stool becomes more difficult for the bowel to move, cramping and pain occur. It most often occurs at the end of the colon, where a majority of the water has been absorbed. Usually constipation can be treated conservatively with oral agents like Miralax, a stool softener. More aggressive treatment with oral laxatives or suppositories (administered rectally) is the next treatment option. Although constipation itself is not dangerous, bowel impactions can occur so badly that normal stool passage does not take place.

The Right Lower Quadrant (RLQ)

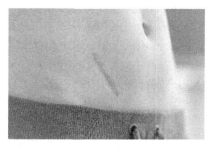

There is one condition that is a must-know in the RLQ: appendicitis. The appendix is a worm-like appendage on the first part of the large intestine called the cecum (see Figure 6.8). When inflamed, as in the case of appendicitis, it poses a risk for rupture, abscess formation, or sepsis. Classically, it begins as a vague abdominal pain somewhat in the middle of the abdomen and gradually localizes to the RLQ. With time, it becomes more tender and painful with minor movements. If the history and exam are suggestive of appendicitis, the physician will begin workup with a CBC, a CT or US of the abdomen, or possibly straight to a surgical consult. If the history and exam are NOT suggestive of appendicitis, again the rationale is discussed in the MDM to demonstrate why the abdominal pain was NOT believed to be appendicitis, i.e. "Pt symptoms not believed to be appendicitis due to two weeks of symptoms and nontender RLQ."

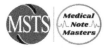

The Epigastrium and RUQ

The upper part of the abdomen called the epigastrium ("epi" = above, "gastrium" = stomach) is one of the more convoluted regions in the abdomen. The underlying anatomical structures include the esophagus, stomach, small intestine (the duodenum), pancreas, liver, and gallbladder. Keep in mind that the epigastrium is quite close to the lower chest, so epigastric symptoms may be worked up for cardiac symptoms and conversely, chest pain may be worked up for GI problems.

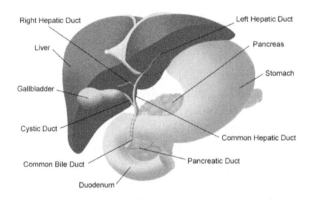

Figure 6.10: Organs and ducts of the epigastrium

Gastroesophageal reflux disease (GERD)

As the name implies, GERD is the reflux of stomach contents up into the esophagus. The stomach is naturally an acidic environment, and GERD often causes a burning-type pain in the epigastrium that may radiate up the mid-chest. Associated symptoms include belching, burping or nausea. GERD symptoms may be alleviated in the short-term by antacids like TUMS, Zantac, or Pepcid, or long-term with proton pump inhibitors (PPI) like omeprazole (Prilosec) taken daily to prevent symptoms. GERD is not generally an urgent concern but is a prevalent cause of upper abdominal and lower chest pain that may warrant workup in the ED to ensure it is not something more serious.

Peptic Ulcer Disease (PUD)

Peptic ulcer disease can develop slowly but may become acute in a matter of days if bleeding occurs. Chronic inflammation, medications, acid, and certain bacteria can lead to erosions of the stomach or intestinal lining, that can develop into an ulcer. An ulcer will cause burning pain in the upper abdomen that may briefly subside after eating (as food absorbs much of the stomach acid) but then returns later when

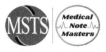

the stomach empties. Many ulcers will heal over time by removing the cause, but deeper ones can erode blood vessels and cause bleeding. As these vessels leak into the digestive tract, the blood is digested and no longer looks like blood, and small amounts are undetectable to the eye (occult). Instead, black, tarry or coffee-ground-like stools called melena can occur, and this is why providers ask seemingly strange questions about stool characteristics. Unfortunately, PUD is not easily imaged in the ED, so the patient may need referral to a gastroenterologist for upper endoscopy (esophagogastroduodenoscopy, or EGD) as an inpatient or an outpatient. Once the acute bleeding is controlled, the patient may be placed on a PPI like omeprazole (Prilosec) or pantoprazole (Protonix) to reduce gastric acid secretion. Oddly, a bacterium *H. pylori* is associated with ulcers, so antibiotics may be required as well.

Cholelithiasis

Cholelithiasis is the formation of mineral stones ("lith" = stone) within the gallbladder ("chole" = bile), colloquially known as gallstones. Gallstones occur in a wide variety of persons and are associated with high-fat diets, obesity, middle-age, and female hormones. These mineral stones may be painful, though benign, if small enough to pass through one of the biliary ducts, which is somewhat similar to kidney stones. If, however, they become lodged and obstruct the flow of bile and other contents into the duodenum, then complications such as cholecystitis or pancreatitis can occur. Gallstones are usually diagnosed through ultrasound, which can detect ~95% of gallstones, and they are sometimes seen on CT scan as well.

Cholecystitis means inflammation ("-itis") of the gallbladder (or bile sac, as "cyst" refers to a fluid-filled sac). If a gallstone obstructs the drainage duct, excessive bile accumulates in the gallbladder, which may lead to inflammation and pain. Because the gallbladder secretes bile in response to fatty foods, this pain classically begins or worsens after eating fatty meals. The pain may wax and wane for a few days, exacerbated by eating, and typically becomes constant once the inflammation becomes more severe. The pain may radiate to the right shoulder blade if the irritation reaches the neighboring tissues.

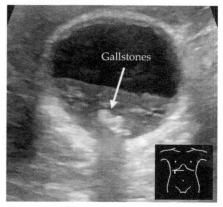

Figure 6.11 Gallbladder ultrasound

Another complication of gallstones is inflammation of the pancreas, called pancreatitis (as you may have predicted). If a gallstone obstructs the pancreatic drainage duct, it leads to inflammation and damage to the pancreatic cells. Pancreatitis is diagnosed with a blood test for lipase, a pancreatic enzyme that breaks down lipids (fats). The pain associated with pancreatitis is typically located in the epigastrium and may radiate to the mid-back. It is generally burning in quality, exacerbated after eating, and is associated with nausea and vomiting. Apart from gallstones, the single most common cause of pancreatitis is excessive chronic alcohol intake, so alcohol intake is a historical element for epigastric abdominal pain.

The Left Upper Quadrant (LUQ)

Luckily the left upper quadrant seldom presents with GI-related problems. The lower rib cage cartilage is prone to inflammation and may present with left, right, or mid epigastric pain, but that is often assessed through simple palpation. The pancreas is also in the LUQ but more posteriorly, so patients less often report LUQ pain as a chief complaint. The kidneys could be considered within the upper quadrants, but they are also anatomically located posteriorly in the flank area.

Figure 6.2: OPQRSTA Comparison of some common abdominal diagnoses

	Peptic Ulcer	Cholecystitis	Pancreatitis
Onset	Gradual	Sudden, stuttering	Varies
Provokers	Empty stomach	Fatty foods	Eating, alcohol
Palliators	Eating	Fasting	Fasting
Quality	Burning	Colicky, sharp	Boring, aching
Radiation	None	Right scapula	Mid-back
Severity	Varies	Varies	Varies
Timing	Constant	Intermittent	Constant
Associated	Melena, weakness, GERD	Nausea, vomiting, diarrhea	Nausea, vomiting
Workup	Occult blood Endoscopy (EGD)	LFTs, ALP US	Lipase CT / ERCP

Considering the relative complexity of the abdominal pain differential diagnosis, it should now be clear why all of the elements of the HPI and exam are so important to document.

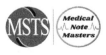

Vaginal Bleeding and Pelvic Pain

Vaginal bleeding is another common ED case that is mostly benign, but with two conditions that elicit concern: significant blood loss and bleeding during pregnancy. Quantifying vaginal bleeding as "heavy" is not always straightforward, as patients may describe the number of pads or tampons, or the number of times pads were changed, or she cannot quantify much at all. Ideally, the number of pads filled in the last 24 hours and the number filled in the last hour 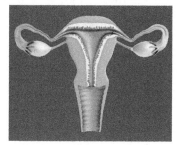 are the numbers sought and recorded. The physician will ask about the patient's last menstrual period (LMP) and other menstrual patterns that could be informative, as well as associated symptoms such as abdominal pain, vaginal discharge, concerns for pregnancy or sexually transmitted infections, etc. Her past medical history will be queried for a history of bleeding disorders, anemia, or anticoagulants.

Reviewing vital signs may reveal signs of significant blood loss, such as tachycardia or hypotension. A pelvic exam is usually required to evaluate for active bleeding, tenderness or discharge, so the patient may be roomed in a special ED room set up for ob/gyn issues. During a pelvic exam, scribes may step behind a privacy curtain or out of the room, and the physician will dictate the findings afterward. By policy, a "chaperone" is often required to remain in the room. The intent of using chaperones is to have a witness that no impropriety occurs during sensitive exams, so if a chaperone was used, document it.

In most non-pregnant patients with vaginal bleeding, as long as vital signs are reassuring and hemoglobin levels are normal, outpatient follow-up is recommended. If the blood count is abnormal, the scribe should pull up previous values for comparison.

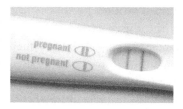

Patients knowingly or unknowingly pregnant present a different situation. Most EDs run a urine pregnancy test on nearly every female who presents with an abdominal or pelvic issue to make sure a surprise pregnancy diagnosis does not occur (and to meet quality metrics covered in a later chapter).

First and foremost, an ectopic pregnancy must be ruled out. "Ectopic" means that the pregnancy is in the wrong place, i.e., not the uterus, and the implantation of a growing embryo in other places can lead to dangerous intra-abdominal bleeding. If a patient has been to a doctor and an intrauterine pregnancy (IUP) has already been confirmed, then we breathe a sigh of relief! If not, a bedside or radiology US is obtained to verify an IUP.

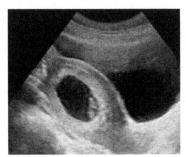

Figure 6.12: Early IUP US. © Nevit Dilmen / CC BY-SA

If the patient has an IUP with bleeding, she is likely concerned about possible miscarriage. Spotting and miscarriages are both common in early pregnancy, but fortunately they are rarely a medical emergency.

Other associated tests the ED physician may order include a blood type and quantitative beta hCG test. Beta hCG (human chorionic gonadotropin) is a hormone produced by the placenta during pregnancy, and in most normal pregnancies the levels increase predictably. The blood type is checked because it can reveal an Rh-incompatibility problem between the mother and embryo that requires additional treatment with medication called RhoGam. An adept scribe will check back in the EHR to see if a blood type is already on file.

Other Pelvic Pain

Pelvic pain, in the absence of pregnancy, can be caused by several factors, including sexually transmitted infections (STIs), endometriosis, and ovarian problems. Most STI test results take a few days to return, so the physician may choose to empirically treat with antibiotics based on the history and exam, rather than wait for the results.

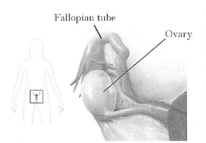

Fallopian tube

Ovary

Figure 6.13: Simple ovarian anatomy Bfpage / CC BY-SA

Ovarian problems such as cysts frequently cause pain from the cyst itself or from cystic fluid that has leaked out causing inflammation. Rarely, an ovary can become twisted around its supporting structures, which compromises blood flow and can lead to ischemia. This condition is called ovarian torsion, and a similar process can occur in testicles. Suspected ovarian pathologies such as these are evaluated with detailed ultrasound in radiology.

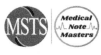

Pyelonephritis and Urolithiasis

The word "pyelonephritis" is the medical term for a kidney infection and can be broken down into roots: "pyelo" = pelvis, the duct connecting the kidney and ureter, "nephr" = kidney, and "itis" = inflammation.

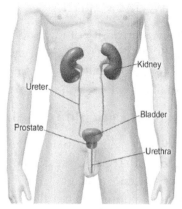

Figure 6.14: Simple male urinary anatomy, BruceBlaus / CC BY-SA

Urinary infections are usually caused by external bacteria that invade upstream. Hence, they are more likely if urinary flow is decreased or stagnant or if a urinary catheter is in use. Bacteria originating from the perineal area can enter the distal urethra and ascend to the bladder (cystitis), potentially continue upward to the kidney (pyelonephritis), or even spread systemically (formerly known as urosepsis).

Simple bladder infections can be treated in clinic, but may present to the emergency room as well. They are characterized by symptoms like urinary urgency, frequency, dysuria (painful urination) or alterations in the color and odor of the urine. In the elderly nursing home population, UTIs may lack classic symptoms, and may possibly be associated with behavioral alterations like confusion.

On exam, patients with pyelonephritis may demonstrate costovertebral angle (CVA) tenderness, since inflammation of the kidney and surrounding tissue will cause pain to percussion in this region. The physician will obtain a urinalysis (UA) and often urine culture to evaluate what type of bacteria is growing in the urine. If an infection is found, antibiotics are administered, and the patient may be sent home or admitted depending on severity.

Urolithiasis is the medical term for kidney stones ("uro" = urine and "lith" = stone). These are caused by the crystallization of dissolved minerals in the urine and are generally benign. However, if this jagged stone moves with urine flow into the narrow, sensitive ureter, it causes exquisite pain and associated nausea. The scraping along the ureter lining can cause microscopic or grossly visible blood in the urine, seen on UA. Pain migrates and severity fluctuates as the stone continues its passage, or symptoms may be constant if the stone is lodged. Most stones will pass on their own or with some help of a medication like tamsulosin (Flomax). Kidney stones can more rarely need urgent treatment if they completely block urine flow.

Low Back Pain

The vast majority of low back pain is attributable to non-emergent musculoskeletal problems. Musculoskeletal causes of back pain tend to be short-lived and are caused by a strain of the muscles or a sprain of the vertebral ligaments. ER management usually involves pain control and further outpatient referrals.

Lumbar radiculopathy and sciatica

Radicular nerve pains are a bit different. The compression of a nerve root can result in lumbar radiculopathy—pain that radiates down one of the legs. When it affects the sciatic nerve, a bundle of nerves (L4-S3), then it is called sciatica, and pain typically radiates from the buttock to the foot. Recall the straight leg raise from the physical exam section, which is performed to elicit these symptoms.

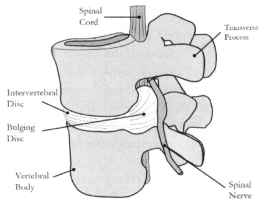

Figure 6.15: Vertebral anatomy with bulging disc

While uncommon, severe compression of the nerve root can lead to loss of nerve function in addition to pain. The pressure needs to be surgically alleviated urgently before the nerve loses its function permanently. The lower extremity neurologic physical exam to test for muscle strength may be limited by pain initially, but needs to be performed before the patient leaves to verify nerve function is uncompromised.

Cauda equina syndrome

Cauda equina means "horsetail," and it refers to the tail-like appearance of the spinal cord in the sacral region. In this region, nerves control bowel and bladder function as well as perineal sensation. Compression of the cauda equina nerves can result in chronic paralysis of the legs, long-term loss of bowel or bladder function, and sexual dysfunction, so this is considered a surgical emergency. To rule out this emergency, the physician may ask some seemingly odd questions regarding incontinence and perineal numbness if cauda equina is a concern. A physical exam of the perineal area for sensation, along with a rectal exam to evaluate muscle tone may also seem odd but are required if these questions or other elements raise suspicion.

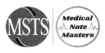

Neurological Emergencies

The neurologic system is incredibly complex and is prone to an array of disorders. We will focus on two main categories of presentations: focal deficits and generalized altered mental status (AMS). AMS is a catch-all chief complaint indicating that the patient's mental state is not right, either in a subtle or severe way, and is often encountered in the elderly population. The history and physical exam are limited, which means clinical logic has little to digest. Glancing at the number of possibilities in Table 6.2 will give you some idea why your provider may need to order a wide range of tests to narrow down AMS possibilities.

Table 6.2: Some common causes of AMS

Stroke	Encephalopathy	Tumor/Mass	Seizure
Dementia	Med Side Effect	Hypoglycemia	Hypothyroidism
Alcohol	Other drugs	Meningitis	Infections
Psychiatric	Opioids	Trauma	Encephalitis

Strokes and intracranial hemorrhage represent two of the most worrisome underlying causes of acute focal neurological issues in the ER, so these will be among the top risky conditions to be ruled out. In the brain, every anatomic region has a function, so the location of blocked blood supply should correlate with functional impairment of that area and should produce correlative symptoms.

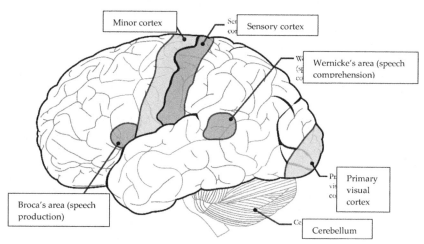

Figure 6.16: Functional landmarks of the cerebrum

176

Figure 6.16 highlights some major cerebral areas that can be affected or impaired by stroke. Broca's area is involved in the expression or articulation of speech, and Wernicke's area is involved in language processing. You could see how damage to these areas might make acquiring the history quite tricky, so instead, we must document those functional deficits in the history and exam.

The cerebellum processes coordination, precision, and timing of movements so damage here can lead to drunk-like discoordination. The motor cortex is responsible for the planning and execution of voluntary movements and the sensory cortex processes touch, pain and other physical sensations. As the name suggests, the visual cortex handles visual data, even though it is on the opposite side from the eyes.

Stroke, Cerebrovascular Accident (CVA)

	Score
Questions on month and age	
0=Answers both correctly, Alert	
1=Answers one correctly	☐
2=Answers neither correctly	
Commands (Eyes opening and hand grip)	
0=Performs both tasks correctly	
1=Performs one task correctly	☐
2=Performs neither task	
Gaze	
0=Normal	
1=Partial gaze palsy	☐
2=Total gaze palsy	
Visual fields	
0=No visual loss	
1=Partial hemianopsia	☐
2=Complete hemianopsia	
3=Bilateral hemianopsia	
Left arm motor	
0=No drift	
1=Drift before 10 seconds	
2=Falls before 10 seconds	☐
3=No effort against gravity	
4=No movement	
Right arm motor	
0=No drift	
1=Drift before 10 seconds	
2=Falls before 10 seconds	☐
3=No effort against gravity	
4=No movement	
Left leg motor	
0=No drift	
1=Drift before 5 seconds	
2=Falls before 5 seconds	☐
3=No effort against gravity	
4=No movement	
Right leg motor	
0=No drift	
1=Drift before 5 seconds	
2=Falls before 5 seconds	☐
3=No effort against gravity	
4=No movement	
Sensory	
0=Normal	☐
1=Abnormal	
Language	
0=Normal	
1=Mild aphasia	☐
2=Severe aphasia	
3=Mute or global aphasia	
Neglect	
0=Normal	
1=Mild	☐
2=Severe	
Modified NIHSS	☐☐

Figure 6.17: Modified NIH Stroke Scale

A stroke or CVA is caused by an interruption of the blood supply to an area of the brain, which deprives brain cells of oxygen and can result in cell death. If the blood supply interruption is transient, causing symptoms temporarily that then remit, it is aptly termed a transient ischemic attack (TIA). In patients presenting with neurological symptoms worrisome for stroke, the physical exam will be heavily focused on the neurological section and may include the NIH stroke scale. Scoring of the stroke scale provides a more standardized approach and further guides treatment decisions. In acute cases, hospitals may have a "stroke protocol," much like a "code STEMI" that is triggered by the score, the precise time of onset, and other factors. Medications to dissolve blood clots and restore blood flow are available, but very

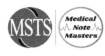

risky because they also dissolve "good" clots, so they are only given if the patient meets all of the current guidelines of the stroke protocol.

After basic care like IV, monitors, and blood work, a patient may receive a head CT or MRI. Standard CTs are better at showing bleeding than ischemia, so specialized CTs or an MRI is often required to identify ischemic areas more accurately. Neurons display minimal regrowth after injury, especially late in life, so many stroke victims will have residual hemiparesis, speech problems, or other deficits that we aim to prevent with aggressive diagnosis and treatment.

Thrombotic ischemic strokes
Thrombotic ischemic strokes are similar to the process of CAD, where blood vessels suffer damage over time due to systemic risk factors. Vessels become less capable of providing consistent blood supply, and narrowed vessels are more likely to become clogged with tiny clots (thrombi) that form over the damaged blood vessel lining. Because it is due to underlying widespread blood vessel damage and aging, multiple blood vessels are affected, and a variety of downstream neurologic symptoms can occur subtly and intermittently. A Transient Ischemic Attack (TIA) is one of these episodes, where blood supply is temporarily insufficient but comes back over time as the small clot naturally dissolves. People refer to this as a "mini-stroke," which is not entirely accurate, but a TIA is indeed a warning of a CVA to come. Thrombotic strokes are more common in the elderly and can be tough to diagnose.

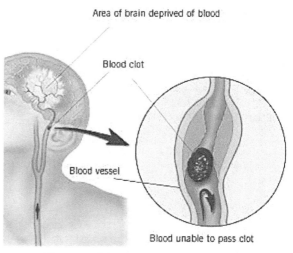

Figure 6.18 Schematic of thrombotic CVA

Hemorrhagic strokes
Hemorrhagic strokes are also associated with damaged blood vessels, but instead of becoming clogged, they rupture – causing bleeding into the adjacent brain tissue. Weakened cerebral vessels may form what is called an aneurysm; a small out-pocketing sometimes described as a "berry." Long-standing hypertension and genetic factors contribute to the formation of aneurysms, and patients may have an

aneurysm for years without knowing it. Because it causes bleeding, a hemorrhagic CVA is also a form of intracranial hemorrhage (see below).

Embolic strokes

Embolic strokes are also caused by a blood vessel becoming clogged, this time by an embolic clot. Recall from the PE segment that an embolus is something that starts in one location but moves elsewhere. In this case, it is not a DVT, but a small clot from the heart or neck. This may seem like an unusual occurrence, but there is one widespread condition that increases the risk of clotting within the heart: atrial fibrillation or "afib." Atrial fibrillation is an irregularly irregular heart rhythm, meaning there is no pattern between heartbeats. When the atria contract in an irregular, uncoordinated manner, blood flow is turbulent and may have stagnant areas that promote thrombus formation. Then, the clot can travel up into the cerebral vessels causing an embolic stroke. Because of the known risk for stroke, patients with afib are placed on an anticoagulant ("blood thinner") like warfarin (Coumadin) or other newer agents like Xarelto and Eliquis.

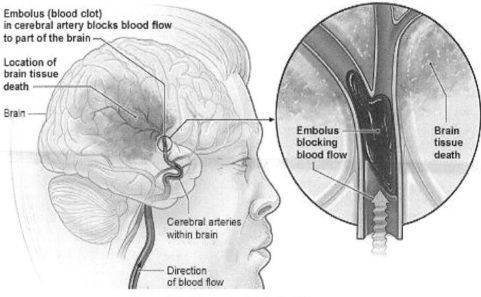

Figure 6.19: Schematic of embolic CVA

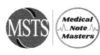

Intracranial Hemorrhage (ICH)

Even a small amount of bleeding within the skull is quite dangerous and causes headache and/or neurologic symptoms. Intracranial bleeds are classified by their location on CT scan—such as subarachnoid (SAH), subdural (SDH), intraparenchymal (IPH) and epidural hemorrhages. ICH can occur following trauma, aneurysm rupture, or with minor triggers in persons on anticoagulants. The presence of blood within the confined space of the cranium causes inflammation, then swelling the local brain tissue and causing neurological symptoms and signs. In cases of head trauma, the physician will also look for signs of a skull fracture. Raccoon eyes (purple bruising beneath the eyes), Battle's sign (bruising behind the ear), and hemotympanum (blood behind the eardrum) are all signs of a skull fracture and possible intracranial hemorrhage.

Table 6.3: Comparison of emergent neurologic events

	Embolic CVA	Thrombotic CVA	Hemorrhagic CVA	Intracranial hemorrhage
Etiology	Embolic clot	Susceptible vessel, thrombus	Aneurysmal or damaged vessel, anticoagulants	Head trauma, aneurysm, anticoagulants
Risk factors	Afib, structural heart issues	Age, HTN, DM, smoking	Age, HTN, DM, smoking, genetics	Anticoagulation, aneurysm genetics
Physical exam	NIH stroke scale including cranial nerve exam, peripheral motor weakness, coordination, speech, cognition			GCS, full neuro exam, possible skull fracture
Treatment	Aspirin, tPA, others	Aspirin, tPA, another anticoagulant	⬇BP, possible aneurysm repair	⬇ pressures, reverse anticoagulants

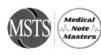

Headaches (HA)

The vast majority of headaches are self-limited and benign, but dangerous conditions like ICH still require rule-out in the ED. Clinical rationale alone may be sufficient, or diagnostic studies may also be needed. In the history, providers will assess for "red flag" symptoms associated with dangerous HA etiologies:

- Neurologic issues (e.g., confusion, motor weakness, sensory changes)
- Vision changes like double vision or loss of vision
- Fever or infectious symptoms
- Medical history, including long-term use of anticoagulants (blood thinners), cancer, or weakened immune defenses
- Sudden, severe onset of headache
- History of head trauma or concussion
- Unusually elevated blood pressure
- A "new" or "different" headache unlike any other

There are three main types of primary headaches – migraine, tension, and cluster. Commonly seen in the ED, migraines are characterized by recurrent headaches with associated nausea, vomiting, light sensitivity (photophobia), sound sensitivity (phonophobia), visual changes like an aura, or cognitive disturbances. "Complex" migraines can even produce stroke-like neurologic symptoms like dysarthria that can trigger a full neurological workup.

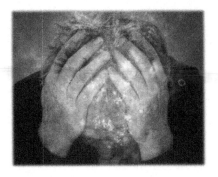

Patients with known migraines present to the ED if they cannot manage their symptoms or if home medications are not working. ED treatment options include anti-inflammatory medications like ketorolac (Toradol) and antiemetics (medications that prevent vomiting, like Reglan). Since migraines are believed to be caused by blood vessel dilation in the brain, medications that constrict blood vessels can be helpful, including triptans (such as Imitrex/ sumatriptan) and caffeine. Opioids are out of favor but are still occasionally used.

Headache workup is directed by the history and physical and will sometimes include a head CT to evaluate for hemorrhage, mass, or other etiologies. More rarely, a lumbar puncture ("spinal tap") is required to detect infections such as meningitis.

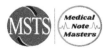

Alcohol Intoxication and Drug Use

Excessive alcohol consumption can have significant health effects, including pancreatitis, hypertension, stroke, hepatitis, liver fibrosis and cirrhosis. In the short-term, excessive alcohol consumption leads to altered mental status with which most people are familiar, but more toxic levels may lead to severe alcohol intoxication, colloquially called "alcohol poisoning."

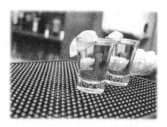

Some common symptoms of acute alcohol intoxication include nausea, vomiting, slowed or irregular breathing, aspiration, decreased body temperature, unconsciousness, and even seizure. Alcohol is undoubtedly the most common drug presenting with problems in the ER, but other drugs such as heroin, cocaine, methamphetamine, LSD, and countless others may be involved as well.

Patients presenting with altered mental status related to acute alcohol and/or drug intoxication are expected to be poor historians, so limitations in the HPI should be documented. Generally, the physician will rely on sober individuals who are familiar with the situation (family, friends, EMS, or the police) to get a clearer idea of the story, and any third-party sources should be specified. For instance, if a paramedic reports that the patient drank a fifth of vodka, the medical note should add "Per EMS," or "EMS reports patient consumed a fifth of vodka."

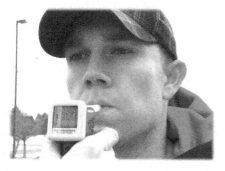

Additionally, it is not uncommon for intoxicated patients to be uncooperative with EMS, police, or the physician when attempting to take a history or perform a physical exam. Patients that acutely pose a danger to themselves or others are placed on a legal "hold" that prohibits them from leaving the controlled environment of the ED until they can demonstrate they are safe. Different states have various terms for a medical hold, but the scribe simply needs to be able to document that a medical hold was placed or lifted. Patients attempting to flee or harm others in the room by thrashing about or striking staff may require security guard assistance, or they may even need to be confined to a gurney using restraints or confined to a locked room. The use of restraints of any sort is a medicolegally hazardous area that requires crystal-clear documentation in the chart.

The physician will examine the patient for any signs of life-threatening injuries as best able and may need to order a blood alcohol content or level (BAC, BAL), drug testing, or other blood tests like a BMP to check for other underlying problems. If the physician believes it is safe, the patient can be dispositioned to detox or home with responsible family members. Alternatively, the physician may calculate the approximate time it will take for the patient to sober up enough to be reexamined and go home independently.

Suicidal Ideation

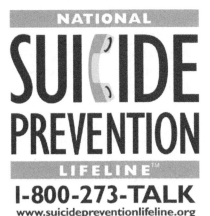

In 2017, over 47,000 people took their own lives, and suicide was the 10th leading cause of death in the US. It is an unfortunate reality that there is an even greater number of people contemplating suicide, and these thoughts are medically termed "suicidal ideation." When a patient presents to the ED with suicidal ideation, either voluntarily or involuntarily, the physician must evaluate the risk of the patient actually harming him/herself. This can be a difficult task given that the physician is likely meeting the patient for the first time, and very personal issues are difficult to discuss in an uncomfortable and fast-paced environment. The patient may not even cooperate with questioning at all. That being said, there are key factors in a patient's story that can inform the physician's clinical decision making. These factors include having a plan to carry out the act, a history of suicide attempts, family history of mental health disease, life stressors, and lack of a social support structure.

After the initial conversation with the patient, the patient may be placed on a medical hold if he or she is not already, and the documentation should make it clear which elements of the history informed this legal decision. The physician will consult with a mental health professional on call, who will in turn speak with the patient in person or via a telemedicine consult. This process often involves a lengthy wait and the patient may wait over multiple shifts. Following the psychology consultation, the patient may be discharged to a safe environment or admitted to a psychiatric facility for further treatment. Many psychiatric facilities have a number of requirements regarding workup and documentation that must be completed before the patient is accepted at their facility.

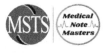

Trauma

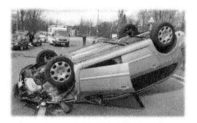

Managing trauma patients is one of the primary reasons emergency departments developed, and you will likely see many trauma patients as an ED scribe. Traumatic injuries can vary from minor local wounds to complicated injuries affecting multiple organ systems. A critical aspect of trauma care is stabilizing a patient and if necessary, transfer to a facility equipped for emergent trauma care (Level One).

One of the most common causes of traumatic injuries is a motor vehicle accident or motor vehicle collision (MVA, MVC). An MVC can cause multiple injuries, and rapid identification of what injuries exist and which are life-threatening is the first step. Then, treatment of these in order of priority must occur quickly, since research shows the majority of deaths occur at the scene of the trauma or within a few hours of arrival to a trauma care facility. Given this, preparedness is essential for treating trauma patients, and EMS may radio ahead to provide some forewarning. As a scribe, the initial report EMS gives is crucial to incorporate in the note. Once the patient arrives and multiple staff converge to provide care, you may be to the side, continuously noting updates on VS, procedures and exam findings on a paper or EHR form. Multiple procedures may occur (each of which requires individual documentation in procedure format) and multiple personnel may call out findings to you for documentation. This is not the time for a scribe to be off your game! To begin the trauma assessment, the physician performs a primary survey that can be remembered as the ABCs of trauma care: Airway, Breathing, and Circulation.

Airway

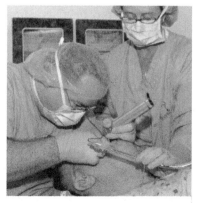

If the airway is obstructed or compromised, this must be identified and rectified immediately, so the airway is the #1 priority. If the airway is compromised by trauma or neurologic defect, the physician may need to insert a tube through the mouth into the trachea to secure the upper airway. Rapid sequence intubation (RSI) is the term for a sequence of preoxygenation, administration of sedative and paralytic medications, then intubation. Once intubated, placement is confirmed and a ventilatory device is attached.

Figure 6.20: Orotracheal intubation

`Date, Time` Procedure Note, Endotracheal Intubation
Performed by: self *(procedures by residents/students require an attending supervisory note)*
Indication: respiratory failure, airway protection
Consent: emergent, patient obtunded
Meds given: 20 mg Etomidate, 150 mg succinylcholine, 1 mg Versed
Procedure: Patient in the supine sniffing position, IV and monitor in place. Preoxygenation via BVM was provided for 3-5 minutes. Rapid sequence induction was provided by administration of 20 mg of Etomidate and 150 mg of Succinylcholine. After generalized fasciculations were noted, a Macintosh laryngoscope was used to directly visualize the vocal cords. A 7.5 mm endotracheal tube was visualized advancing between the cords to a level of 23 cm at the teeth. The stylet was then removed and syringe aspiration performed with reassuring result. Tube placement was also noted by fogging in the tube, equal and bilateral breath sounds, no sounds over the epigastrium, and end-tidal colorimetric monitoring. The cuff was then inflated with 10cc's of air and the tube secured. A good pulse oximetry wave form was seen on the monitor throughout the procedure. The patient was then connected to the ventilator with settings per respiratory. A portable chest x-ray has been ordered for placement. Continued sedation will be provided by Propofol continuous infusion titrated to a Ramsay score of 2 to 3. The patient tolerated the procedure well.
Complications: none

Breathing and ventilation

Breathing or ventilation is the movement of air in and out of the lungs. VS such as RR, O2 sats +/- carbon dioxide levels are indicators of ventilation efficacy, and poor ventilation may need assistance with bag-valve masks, positive-pressure ventilation masks, or a ventilator for intubated patients.

Circulation

During this step, cardiac pump effectiveness and sources of blood loss are identified. Hypotension and tachycardia are indicators of circulatory compromise, and the patient may require several peripheral iv's or a large central iv to be placed for fluids or blood administration. ED physicians perform what is called a FAST exam (Focused Assessment with Sonography for Trauma) that quickly screens for the presence of abdominal fluid.

In addition to the ABCs, "D" and "E" are often included as discussed next.

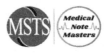

Disability (neurologic)

A neurologic exam is performed for suspected head trauma, including the Glasgow Coma Scale (GCS), which evaluates the patient's motor, verbal, and eye responses. The responses are scored from 3 to 15 (normal function) according to the chart below. When dictating the physical exam, the ED physician may say something like "GCS 14" or may specify each category.

Table 6.4: The Glasgow Coma Scale (GCS)

Response	Scale	Points
Eye opening response	eyes open spontaneously	4 points
	eyes open to verbal command, speech, or shouting	3 points
	eyes open only to pain	2 points
	no eye opening	1 point
Verbal response	oriented, conversant	5 points
	confused but able to answer questions	4 points
	inappropriate responses but words are discernible	3 points
	incomprehensible sounds or speech	2 points
	no verbal response	1 point
Motor response	obeys commands for movement	6 points
	purposeful movement to a painful stimulus	5 points
	withdraws from pain	4 points
	abnormal (spastic) flexion to pain	3 points
	extensor (rigid) response to pain	2 points
	no motor response	1 point

Exposure

The multiple trauma patient is completely undressed, and the body is examined head-to-toe for signs of injury. EMS often transports trauma patients on a long hard backboard with a neck collar in place, so at some point, the patient must be rolled to examine the dorsum for injury. After the scan for injuries is complete, additional tests, including essential lab tests or an EKG, may be performed. Since alcohol use and trauma often coincide, the ER may perform blood alcohol testing for medical and/or legal purposes, and police may be present.

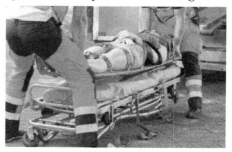

Figure 6.21: EMS backboard and C-collar

There are many other types of trauma (gunshot wounds, assaults, and falls) that we do not cover but follow the same general guidelines. In some cases, the documentation of these visits may be used later for legal purposes.

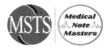

Dental Pain

Patients often present to the emergency department with dental pain if the pain is unmanageable or if they are unable to see a dentist quickly. According to the American Dental Association, emergency departments have seen a dramatic increase in dental pain patients, from 1.1 million in 2000 to 2.2 million in 2012, but 80% of those visits are due to preventable conditions. While the ED physician will inform the patient that following up with a dentist or oral surgeon is needed for definitive care, the ED physician can help the patient with dental pain in the meantime.

A dental block, or alveolar nerve block, is a tried-and-true ED treatment for dental pain. An injection of local anesthetic such as lidocaine to the area of the alveolar nerve blocks pain sensation from the lower teeth. If you have ever had teeth pulled or filled, this is the shot you received to be numbed before the procedure. Ideally, patients experience hours of relief until they can see a dentist or oral surgeon. Topical benzocaine mixtures are also useful, such as Orajel. During the physical exam, the ED physician will palpate the face for facial swelling, palpate the teeth and gums for tenderness or swelling, and may percuss the teeth to assess for sensitivity. If the dental pain is due to significant facial trauma, the ED physician may assess for a mandibular fracture by asking the patient to bite down hard upon a wooden tongue depressor. The physician may note findings as "right lower rear molars," or you may need to record the more formal tooth number(s) in the physical exam, as shown in Figure 4.3.

Dental infections are common causes of pain. Generally speaking, a dental infection occurs when oral bacteria invade part of the tooth that is damaged or decayed. This can result in a pus collection around the tooth's root, known as a periapical abscess. Abscesses can be quite painful, but fortunately the ED physician can cut open (incise) the abscess and drain the pus in a procedure called an incision and drainage (I&D). I&D procedures are frequent in the ED, in many different locations.

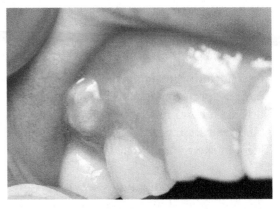

Figure 6.22: Dental abscess

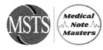

Complex Patients

Most of the visits discussed in this chapter have been addressed as singular pathologies, but in real life, patients often have multiple coexisting medical and psychological issues at play. For example, a patient with a chief complaint of cough could be seemingly simple. However, after seeing the patient, we learn the patient has a long-standing history of smoking, asthma, COPD, and coronary artery disease, and suddenly the complexity has significantly increased. All of these relevant histories need to be included, and not only will they increase the complexity, but they will change how a provider will treat the cough. As a scribe, careful documentation of the A&P will make it clear why the provider would choose to manage a healthy 19-year-old differently than the patient above.

Another instance of increased complexity is what might initially appear to be a medication refill. While these visits can be straightforward, multiple medications mean multiple underlying medical problems. A patient with hypertension, anxiety, and diabetes may not even remember all of his/her medications and may be experiencing side effects.

Common Emergency Medicine Medications

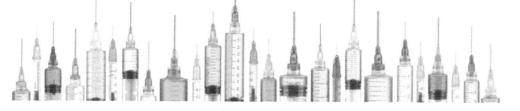

This section will introduce some of the most commonly-encountered medications in the emergency department. You do not need to understand the pharmacology at this point in your career, but if a patient comes into the ED and nitroglycerin is in their medication list, then you should instantly suspect that he/she has a history of coronary artery disease. So, it should be your goal to remember the primary indication for each medication, whether that is analgesia (pain relief), hypertension, etc. Note that the format for naming drugs is to put the generic name first, followed by the capitalized brand name in parentheses (e.g., ondansetron (Zofran)). The generic name is generally preferred and should be spelled correctly. If you cannot understand a medication name said by the provider, it is best to insert a placeholder such as *** into the note for the provider to complete later, rather than write a medication name that is inaccurate.

Table 6.4: Common ED medications and descriptions

Medication	Description
Acetaminophen (Tylenol)	an analgesic and antipyretic (fever reducer)
Albuterol (Ventolin, Proventil)	Bronchodilator used in inhalers and nebulizers to open airways in asthma, wheezing or allergic reactions. Sometimes combined with ipratropium (Duoneb)
Amiodarone	Antiarrhythmic medication used IV to convert afib and other arrythmias
Aspirin	Baby aspirin is used to prevent the risk of heart disease by limiting platelet aggregation, and full-dose aspirin is used in cases of acute chest pain
Azithromycin (Zithromax)	IV or PO antibiotic used for bacterial infections of the respiratory tract and some STIs
Ceftriaxone (Rocephin)	IV cephalosporin antibiotic used for a variety of bacterial respiratory and GU tract infections
Cephalexin (Keflex)	Oral antibiotic for skin infections
Ciprofloxacin (Cipro)	Oral or IV antibiotic for GI and GU infections
Clopidogrel (Plavix)	Similar to aspirin, Plavix inhibits platelet aggregation and is used for coronary and cerebral vessel disease
Dextrose or D50	Dextrose is similar to glucose and is used IV for hypoglycemia
Digoxin (Lanoxin)	From the foxglove plant, digoxin is an antiarrhythmic used for many years, but falling out of favor
Diphenhydramine (Benadryl)	an oral or parenteral antihistamine that reduces symptoms of swelling and pruritis in allergic reactions
Epinephrine ("epi")	I.e. adrenaline, epinephrine is used IV in cardiac arrest and anaphylaxis, and SQ with anesthetics like lidocaine
Furosemide (Lasix)	Diuretic used to treat congestive heart failure (CHF)
GI cocktail	A combination of Maalox, lidocaine +/- donnatal given for epigastric pain as a fast-acting local pain reliever

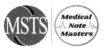

Haldol	An antipsychotic used IM to control agitated behavior. Olanzapine is similarly used.
Heparin, low-molecular weight heparin (LMWH)	Parenteral anticoagulants used to treat thrombi such as DVT and PE and acute coronary syndrome
Hydrochlorothiazide (HCTZ)	Diuretic (increases urine output) used to treat HTN
Ibuprofen (Advil, Motrin)	An NSAID used to reduce pain and inflammation
Insulin	The hormone that acts to lower blood sugars and is used to treat hyperglycemia in type I and type II diabetes mellitus. Generally fast-acting insulin types are used in an ED such as aspartate (Novolog) or lispro (Humalog).
Lidocaine	Anesthetic applied topically or injected to block nerve sensation for pain relief. Bupivacaine is similar.
Lisinopril	an angiotensin-converting enzyme (ACE) inhibitor that treats high blood pressure
Lorazepam (Ativan)	In the benzodiazepine class, it is used to treat anxiety states, alcohol withdrawal, seizures, and sedation for procedures. Diazepam (Valium) is similar.
Metformin	First-line medication for type II diabetes that increases a person's sensitivity to insulin
Metoprolol	The most common beta-blocker, which reduces blood pressure and slows heart rate, most commonly for hypertension and CHF
polyethylene glycol 3350 (MiraLAX)	Stool softener taken to relieve constipation or prepare for colonoscopy
Naloxone (Narcan)	Medication that ANtagonizes NARCotics, used to treat opioid overdose
Nitroglycerin or ntg	Medication used to sublingually, IV or topically dilate blood vessels in coronary artery disease
Omeprazole (Prilosec)	Proton-pump inhibitor that reduces gastric acid production. Protonix is similar but can be given IV.
Ondansetron (Zofran)	Common medication used to alleviate nausea either sublingually or IV

Penicillin (Pen Vee-K, Bicillin)	Oral, IV or IM medication now most often used for strep throat. Bicillin is a long-acting IM shot.
Phenergan	Anti-emetic medication with some sedative properties, also used for vertigo
Phenytoin (Dilantin)	Mainstay medication for epilepsy
Prednisone	Anti-inflammatory steroids with myriad uses including asthma, allergic reactions, swelling
sumatriptan (Imitrex)	Migraine medication in the -triptan class. Rizatriptan and zolmitriptan are similar.
Vancomycin	IV antibiotic for resistant bacteria
Warfarin (Coumadin)	Anti-coagulant taken daily by patients with a history or risk of forming blood clots, and tested with INR lab

In addition to the medications above, stronger pain relievers are often needed in an ER setting. Injuries may warrant IV/IM or oral opioids acutely, with a short prescription for home to be used until the patient can follow up. Opioid pain medications have come under increased scrutiny due to their potential for long-term dependence, abuse, and overdose, and some states require that before prescribing an opioid, the physician must consult a prescription drug registry that logs all the patient's controlled substance prescriptions throughout the state. Even if not required, this practice gives the ED physician valuable information about the patient's prescriptions, and you should document if the physician does this review and what was found.

Table 6.6: Common opioid medications and their use in the ED

Medication	Description
morphine	Standard IV medication used for acute pain relief
hydromorphone (Dilaudid)	Available in oral and IV forms, an alternative to morphine
fentanyl	Potent IV opioid, but shorter-acting
hydrocodone (Norco)	oral only, combined with Tylenol
oxycodone (Percocet)	oral only, combined with Tylenol
Tramadol (Ultram)	Oral pain reliever with semi-opioid effects

Making flashcards may help you memorize these, and you will find yourself familiar with these and many other medications after several ED shifts.

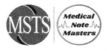

A Complete Note Example

You have now read a great deal about medical documentation, but it may be difficult to imagine how all of these elements come together coherently. To put everything together, review the following examples of a complete note from start to finish.

CC: facial lac

HPI: Eric Little is a healthy 8 y/o M who presents to the ER with a facial laceration. Incident occurred approximately 1 h PTA, when he tripped and hit his face against the edge of a coffee table. No LOC. Mother heard a bump and he yelled immediately afterward. She reports he has been acting normally after the incident, aside from initial fear reacting to the blood. No other injuries. Last po intake 2 h PTA.

ROS:
Constitutional: No fever or recent illness
Eyes: Denies vision or hearing changes
GI: denies n/v
Neuro: Denies extremity paresthesia

Allergies: Penicillin (rash)
Medications: ranitidine prn

Past Medical History: GERD, seasonal allergies
Fully immunized per mother
Social History: parents divorced. Lives primarily at home with mother, visits father every other weekend. Dad smokes, but always outside.

Physical Exam:
Vital Signs: HR: 90, RR: 20, Oximetry: 99% RA Weight: 57 lbs (25.8kg)
GENERAL: Patient is pleasant, well-nourished, active, no acute distress.
HEENT: Normocephalic. External canals and TMs wnl. Nose atraumatic. Oropharynx wnl. No conjunctival injection or icterus. PERRL, EOMI.
NECK: full ROM, nontender.
RESPIRATORY: Lungs are CTA without wheeze or rhonchi. Good air movement.
CARDIOVASCULAR: Regular rate and rhythm. No murmurs, rubs, or gallops.

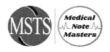

NEUROLOGIC: Awake, alert, interactive. Facial movements symmetric. Eyebrow raise and smile symmetric. Facial sensation intact peripheral to injury.
PSYCHIATRIC: Normal cognition and speech for age, interacting well with mom
SKIN: scattered 1-2 cm round ecchymosis on anterior lower legs, otherwise no other external signs of trauma.

> Facial skin reveals obliquely oriented full-thickness laceration overlying the R outer orbit, 3.8 cm in length, with protruding SQ adipose. Medial aspect intrudes 1 cm into eyebrow hair, but without obvious hair follicle loss. No active bleeding. Mild surrounding swelling without tissue maceration.

ED Course:
1400 Pt roomed in room 6. LET placed from triage, some blanching already present.
d/w mom possibility of sedation for the procedure, but would prefer to avoid.
1445 Wound prepped and repair begun.
1530 Pt reassessed, doing well, having a snack. Behavior normal per mom.

Procedure Note: Laceration repair, Intermediate Layered Closure
Indication: R facial laceration, 3.8 cm length
Universal protocol observed with time-out, correct site, and patient confirmed.
Performed by: self
Consent: verbal informed consent obtained from patient and parent
Medications administered: topical LET then 2 mL 1% lidocaine with epi SQ
Procedure: after adequate anesthesia obtained, wound was copiously irrigated with NS then prepped and draped. No FB visible on inspection. Wound depth palpated, no underlying bony abnormalities or FB. Deep layer closed with running 5-O Vicryl, and superficial layer with 6-O Ethilon x 10 simple interrupted sutures with good approximation. Patient was able to raise eyebrow without gaping or focal wound tension. Steri-strips placed over lateral aspect to additionally minimize tension.
Complications: None, pt tolerated well

Assessment & Plan
Healthy 8 y/o M with facial laceration. No LOC and no neuro signs to suggest CHI, has now been 2.5 h since injury, but mom was advised of warning signs including excess sleepiness, n/v, behavior changes, etc. Cosmetic repair achieved, however the inevitability of scarring and possible eyebrow hair growth changes were discussed. Low likelihood of retained FB or wound contamination based on mechanism, but

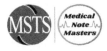

infection is still possible and s/s of infection also d/w mom. Abx not routinely prescribed since side effects outweigh possible benefit.

Dx: facial laceration without foreign body initial visit S01.XA

Plan:
1. Keep wound clean and dry. Steri-strips will fall off on their own.
2. f/u with PCP for suture removal in 5 days
3. Some scarring is unavoidable, but avoiding UV exposure, avoiding picking or itching can minimize scar
4. Be alert for redness, discharge, swelling or other signs of infection. Seek evaluation with PCP if those arise, and return to ED if unable to be seen quickly.
5. Mom given laceration care handout and voices understanding of the plan

(The repair itself is coded as CPT 12052 based upon the length, complexity, and location, all of which is specified in the procedure note.)

End of Chapter Quiz

1. A "kidney infection" is more technically known as what?
   a. Peptic ulcer disease
   b. Nephrosis
   c. Nephrolithiasis
   d. Pyelonephritis

2. Which condition is NOT typically characterized by epigastric pain?
   a. Peptic ulcer disease
   b. Pancreatitis
   c. Cholelithiasis
   d. Colitis

3. Which lab test is used to diagnose pancreatitis?
   a. Lipase
   b. Alkaline phosphatase (ALP)
   c. D-dimer
   d. Troponin

4. Which of these medications is a risk factor for hemorrhagic stroke?
   a. cephalexin
   b. coumadin
   c. ciprofloxacin
   d. caffeine

5. What is the most common source of clot in a pulmonary embolus?
   a. Appendicitis
   b. Heart atria
   c. DVT
   d. Varicose veins

6. Which lab test can detect trace amounts of myocardial cell death?
   a. Troponin
   b. D-dimer
   c. Hemoglobin
   d. Lipase

7. Acute appendicitis presents with focal pain in which abdominal region?
   a. Right upper quadrant (RUQ)
   b. Left upper quadrant (LUQ)
   c. Left lower quadrant (LLQ)

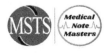

    d. Right lower quadrant (RLQ)

8. Which proton pump inhibitor helps reduce acid secretion in the stomach in patients with PUD?

    a. Zantac

    b. Pantoprazole

    c. Nitroglycerin

    d. Hydrochlorothiazide

9. True or False: Abdominal pain that is worse after eating fatty foods is concerning for cholelithiasis.

    a. True

    b. False

10. Which lab test helps detect the presence of a blood clot?

    a. D-dimer

    b. Troponin

    c. Lipase

    d. ALP

11. PE and stroke from atrial fibrillation are both caused by embolism.

    a. True

    b. False

12. This is acceptable procedure documentation: Physician performed FAST exam and no intra-abdominal fluid was seen.

    a. True

    b. False

13. If a patient denies seeing blood in the stool, a GI bleed is not possible.

    a. True

    b. False

Answers: 1. D 2. D 3. A 4. B 5. C 6. A 7. D 8. B 9. B 10. A 11. A 12. B 13. B

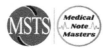

7. Billing and Reimbursement

Accurate and comprehensive documentation of each visit ensures fair compensation to the department, as well as the individual provider. A good scribe captures these details, and in turn, further justifies the scribe service expense. Medical billing and coding is a complex topic that few healthcare providers know much about, or maybe even *want* to know much about. However, knowledge deficits in this area can have long-term ramifications for physicians who fail to learn how to capture revenue. Leaving money on the table is inefficient and may just lead to more work in the long-run, so thorough documentation with billing parameters in mind captures the reimbursement that is due and improved efficiency reduces long-term workload.

We will walk through the process so that you have an idea of how your note will be analyzed, which will help you build useful templates. After a visit, signed medical notes are submitted to a billing and coding company who assigns numeric codes to the visit based on the quality and complexity of the documentation, as well as any procedures performed. In the past, the billing specialist was a human being, but now EHRs have background billing and coding programming that semi-automates the process. Artificial intelligence-based computer-assisted-coding programs have also been developed to analyze the text of the note and improve coding accuracy with fewer human hours required.

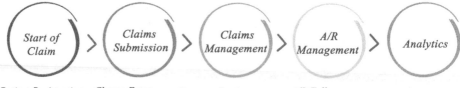

Start of Claim	Claims Submission	Claims Management	A/R Management	Analytics
Patient Registration Insurance Eligibility Patient Appointment	Charge Entry Medical Coding	Payment Posting Medical Coding Services Denial Management Appeals	A/R Follow up Patient Collections Patient Statements	

Based on the assigned service codes, a bill is sent to payers like private insurers, Medicare, Medicaid, or self-pay patients. The documentation must support the level of billing, since discrepancies can lead to an incredibly unpleasant audit. Medicare (for the elderly) and Medicaid (for lower incomes) are the two largest government payers and are under the umbrella of Centers for Medicare & Medicaid Services (CMS). This agency sets the standard for reimbursement that many others follow. They also determine Relative Value Unit (RVU), which is a further modification of payment based on estimates of local costs such as malpractice insurance. CMS modifies small regulations frequently, but January 2021 marked

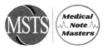

the largest shift in outpatient billing strategy since 1997. Right now, the changes **only** apply to outpatient clinics including most urgent cares, but other venues like the emergency room and inpatient wards may be soon to follow.

Outpatient E/M Levels

An evaluation and management level (E/M level) is the billing term for how complicated the medical evaluation and treatment was for the visit. This level is the primary determinant for how much payers will reimburse, and the numbers range from level 1 to 5. A level 1 is relatively rare, so simple as just getting a flu shot where a physician is not necessarily required. Level 2 could be something like bug bite that needs an OTC cream. Thus, nearly all routine outpatient visits are levels 3, 4, or 5, with levels 3 and 4 as the most commonly billed in primary care clinic.

To charge a given E/M level, specific criteria must be documented within the patient's note. The requirements for a new vs. established patient were slightly different, so some providers are in the habit of mentioning in the first HPI sentence if the patient is new or established. For reference, Table 7.1 outlines the elements previously required. A certain number of elements were counted in the HPI, the ROS, the SHx/FHx/PMHx, the physical exam, and complexity level in the medical decision making. Before 2021, the E/M level was determined by counting the number of elements in each category, sometimes referred to as "bean counting," which was tedious and seemed out-of-touch with clinical care. After many years, the AMA and CMS decided to revamp the E/M billing system for outpatient visits in 2021.

Table 7.1: 1995/1997 E/M levels for established patients (for reference)

Established Patients	Level 1 (99211)	Level 2 (99212)	Level 3 (99213)	Level 4 (99214)	Level 5 (99215)
CC	+	+	+	+	+
HPI (OPQRST)	0	≥ 1	≥ 1	≥ 4	≥ 4
ROS	0	0	≥ 1	≥ 2	≥ 10
PMHx, PSHx, FamHx	0	0	0	1	≥ 2
Physical exam	0	≥1 element	≥1 in affected system + 1-8 others	≥ 12 element ≥ 2 systems	≥ 9 systems
MDM	0	Minimal	Low	Moderate	Complex

Note, the old ROS "bean" counting requirements, which explains in part why the ROS elements listed in Chapter 3 are explained – because it affected billing. The ROS is a good example of the frustration providers encountered with the old fashion of E/M determination, that depended more on beans than the effort, time, or mental energy spent on patient care.

The updated 2021 E/M tables are shown below, and it should be fairly obvious the major differences from Table 7.1. The first major difference is that the E/M level no longer relies upon counting beans in the Subjective and Physical Exam sections. This does not mean that these sections can just be glossed over, however, since the HPI and some elements of the physical exam are essential information going into CDM, and any piece of information that is interpreted in the A&P should first be documented in the Subjective or Objective Sections.

Table 7.2: 2021 E/M levels for new patients

New Patients	Level 2 (99202)	Level 3 (99203)	Level 4 (99204)	Level 5 (99205)
CC				
HPI (OPQRST)				
ROS		"Medically appropriate"		
PMHx, PSHx, FamHx				
Physical exam				
MDM Complexity	Straight-forward	Low	Moderate	High
Time	15-29	30-44	45-59	60-74

Table 7.3: 2021 E/M levels for established patients

New Patients	Level 2 (99212)	Level 3 (99213)	Level 4 (99214)	Level 5 (99215)
CC				
HPI (OPQRST)				
ROS		"Medically appropriate"		
PMHx, PSHx, FamHx				
Physical exam				
MDM Complexity	Straight-forward	Low	Moderate	High
Time	10-19	20-29	30-39	40-54

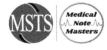

Billing by Time

Alternatively, the E/M level for outpatient visits (not the ER) can be set based on the total time spent with the patient and associated care like reviewing results, tracking down information, making phone calls, etc. By now, you likely realize visits commonly take far longer than expected, so being able to be reimbursed for additional time is a valuable option. Billing by time may also come into play when a provider's focus involves more socioeconomic determinants of health or mental health counseling, that can be time-consuming and would be a low E/M level based on the old bean-counting method.

Table 7.4: Anticipated times for clinic E/M levels

New Patient Visit	Expected time	Established Patient Visit	Expected time
99201	10	99211	5
99202	20	99212	10
99203	30	99213	15
99204	45	99214	25
99205	60	99215	40

Now suppose a family presents with an elderly patient who needs to be admitted to a nursing home. The provider may spend 45 minutes with them, but then a lot of additional time is spent making phone calls and doing paperwork. In this case, the HPI and MDM should be level 5 material, and the extra time spent with the patient can boost what might otherwise be a level 3 to a level 5 if it is appropriately documented. Prior to 2021, the documentation had to specify how much time was spent *face-to-face* with the patient, as opposed to additional time on the phone with the nursing home, reviewing results, etc. In 2021, the requirement is focused on the total time on that calendar date, and that it was the *provider's* time, not general staff:

> *Total time personally spent on comprehensive patient care on this date was 45 minutes, including lab and US review, and consultation with the labor and delivery unit at Sunrise Hospital. Time is exclusive of separately billable procedures.*

Note that separately billable procedures are NOT part of the time, just like they are separate from the E/M level. These cases may be evident to you as they occur, and you can ask your provider if he/she would like the time documented, or you can insert a placeholder into the note.

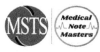

Emergency Department E/M

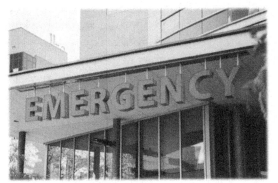

Emergency department E/M levels are similar to outpatient clinics and urgent care conceptually, using elements in each section of the medical note using the older method. Higher E/M levels are more common, however, reflecting the acute care nature of the ER. Scribes should anticipate that a level 5 visit is a common occurrence (sometimes 50% of visits, depending on the local setting), and plan accordingly with documentation templates that would support a level 5 visit. The older "bean counting" approach is **still in effect** for the ER so scribes must be diligent to ensure all the necessary beans are in place.

Table 7.5: 1995-1997 E/M level required elements

	Level 1	Level 2	Level 3	Level 4	Level 5
CC	+	+	+	+	+
HPI (OPQRST)	1-3	1-3	1-3	≥ 4	≥ 4
ROS elements	0	1	1	2-9	≥ 10
Medical, Social, Family histories	0	0	0	≥ 1	≥ 2
Physical exam systems	1	2-7	2-7	2-7	≥ 8
MDM complexity	None	Minimal	Low	Moderate	Complex

Note, no CC = no payment! For this reason, an RFV or CC is required, although it is acceptable to pull forward a CC entered by intake staff.

To set up initial note templates, it is best to just build the template based on level 5 requirements so that you have the required structure laid out, and maximal coding is possible. One trick is in the physical exam, which has to include eight body *systems*, not areas or regions as is acceptable in levels 1-4.

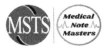

1. Constitutional (e.g. general)	7. Genitourinary
2. Eyes	8. Musculoskeletal
3. Ears, nose, mouth, and throat	9. Skin
4. Cardiovascular	10. Neurologic
5. Respiratory	11. Psychiatric
6. Gastrointestinal	12. Hematologic/lymphatic/immunologic

ED Observation ("Obs")

In addition to levels 1-5, emergency departments may also bill for Observation and Critical Care time. Utilization of the Observation concept varies greatly amongst ERs, depending on physical space, staffing, and admission patterns, but generally accounts for <5% of all visits. A typical Observation visit might be in an ER with ample space, where a patient is able to stay for a prolonged period for reassessments rather than being moved into the main hospital for observation. Observation might be more frequent in newer "standalone" ERs, that are not physically connected to a hospital. Good examples would be an asthma patient that could likely go home after 8 hours of medications and reassessments, or a low-risk chest pain patient that needs serial labs before going home. If your ER utilizes an Observation unit, be sure to use EHR or local templates, since specific documentation is required.

Critical Care Time

If a patient requires truly emergent medical care, such as serious trauma or a possible heart attack or stroke, the physician can be reimbursed for "critical care time," which is conceptually similar to billing by time in the clinic. The American Medical Association defines critical care time as follows:

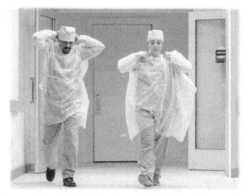

"Critical care is defined as a physician's (or physicians') direct delivery of medical care for a critically ill or critically injured patient. A critical illness or injury acutely impairs one or more vital organ systems such that there is a high probability of imminent or life-threatening deterioration in the patient's condition.

Critical care involves high complexity decision making to assess, manipulate, and support vital system functions to treat single, or multiple, vital organ system failure; and/or to prevent further life-threatening deterioration of the patient's condition."

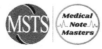

8. Summary

Common problems for which an ED physician may choose to bill for critical care include, but are not limited to:

- Trauma
- Severe infections/sepsis
- Myocardial infarction
- Cardiac arrhythmias
- Stroke
- Respiratory failure
- Acute GI bleeding
- Severe asthma requiring continuous nebulizer treatment

There are some obvious clues as to when critical care time will be billed, since these are usually the visits in the larger critical care bays, and there are multiple staff involved. It may be difficult to know precisely how much time to document, but inserting a phrase into the note as below will signal the physician to fill this in when they review and sign the note:

> *Total critical care time personally spent in the direct care of this patient, excluding separately billable procedures: *** minutes.*

Note that separately billable procedures are NOT part of the time, just like they are separate from the E/M level. Everything else associated with the patient care is included in the total time, just like it is in clinic. Critical care cases may be evident to you as they occur, and you can ask your provider if he/she would like the time documented or you can insert the placeholder into the note.

To get a sense of what is most common in the ED, Table 7.6 lists the twenty most commonly billed items, in order, and their associated codes for 2016, as reported by ACEP, the American College of Emergency Physicians:

Table 7.6: Most commonly billed ED codes

1.	E/M Level IV ED Visit	99284
2.	E/M Level III ED Visit	99283
3.	E/M Level V ED Visit	99285
4.	EKG Rhythm Interpretation with Strip	93042
5.	E/M Level II ED Visit	99282
6.	Single Laceration up to 2.5cm (scalp, neck, axillae, etc.)	12001
7.	Single Laceration up to 2.5cm (face, ears, eyelids, nose, lips)	12011
8.	Application of short leg splint (calf to foot)	29515
9.	Critical Care 1st Hour	99291

10. Single Laceration Repair 2.6 to 7.5cm (scalp, neck, axillae, etc.)	12002
11. Application of Finger Splint	29130
12. Application of Short Arm Splint (forearm to hand)	29125
13. E/M Level I ED Visit	99281
14. Application of Long Leg Splint (thigh to ankle or toes)	29505
15. Treatment of Shoulder Dislocation	23650
16. Spinal Puncture - Lumbar	62270
17. Dressings or Debridement of Partial-Thickness Burns	16020
18. Single Laceration 2.6 up to 5.0cm (face, ears, eyelids, nose, lips)	12013
19. Endotracheal Intubation	31500
20. I&D Abscess Simple/Single	10060

Medical Decision Making in E/M Levels

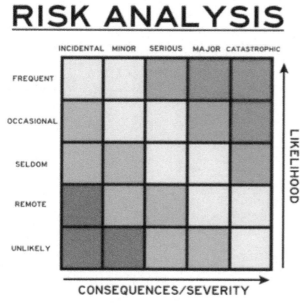

The second large shift in billing method for outpatient visits is an increased focus on medical decision making, which is aligned with what clinicians find most important. So when it comes to the MDM, how do they determine minimal, low, moderate, or complex levels? Essentially, points are given for elements documented in the note that contribute to a patient's overall medical risk and intervention level. As a scribe, these might not be obvious at first, but close observation of the provider's actions and discussions with the patient/staff will help.

The new full MDM scoring grid can be found online, but the take-home points for the documentation assistant are that three main categories of MDM are considered, as described next.

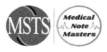

1. **The number of diagnostic and management options**

   After the physician performs the HPI and exam and reviews the chart, the initial impression of the MDM outlines WHY he/she decided to order tests and therapies, but perhaps decided to defer other ones. A straightforward RFV in a healthy patient likely has only a couple options as to what might be ordered for testing and therapy, but more complex patients might have dozens of branches in the decision-making tree.

   - Did the physician consider a number of different diagnoses?
   - Did the physician order a variety of diagnostics to figure out the issue?
   - Did the physician have to think through the risks and benefits of different management options?
   - Did the physician consider ordering a few different types of imaging before selecting the best one for this patient?

2. **The amount and complexity of information analyzed**

   This component addresses how much information the physician needed to review and digest in order to make an assessment.

   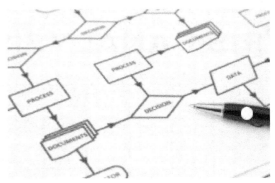

   - Did the physician talk to the radiologist to discuss worrisome findings?
   - Did the physician go back to look at old notes or external records?
   - Did the physician compare today's results to previous ones?
   - Did the physician seek other sources of HPI, like calling family or a nursing home?
   - Was another physician consulted?
   - Did the physician interpret the imaging personally or just read the radiologist's interpretation?
   - Did the physician interpret all of the labs and imaging?

3. **The amount of risk to the patient, and what was done about it**

   This category considers how risky the patient's problem is, and how risky the required medical interventions are. Something that seems initially harmless may turn out to be a dangerous diagnosis after workup and vice versa, so the MDM

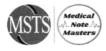

should explain the risk considerations overall. A stubbed toe that will heal on its own would be on one end of the spectrum, since the risk of the diagnosis and the risk of the treatment are both negligible. On the other end of the spectrum would be a cardiac arrest requiring resuscitation and emergent bypass surgery, since both the condition and the treatment are quite risky.

- Is the condition considered self-limited? Worsening? Unstable?
- Did the condition require treatment *during* the visit?
- Did the condition require risky invasive testing?
- Did the condition warrant prescriptions for home, or just OTC?
- Did the patient require admission or transfer?
- Did the patient require a procedure or surgery?
- Did the patient's issue represent significant morbidity or mortality risk?

New for 2021 is consideration of socioeconomic determinants of health, that contribute to the overall treatment prognosis for the patient. Examples would be homelessness, food insecurity, or financial difficulty in acquiring medications. Shown below is an EHR template designed to capture these elements as discrete data clicks, would are designed to help automate counting points.

Figure 7.1: EHR template for click entry of socioeconomic determinants of health

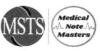

Medical Necessity

The scribe also needs to be generally aware of the concept of medical necessity. A payer receiving a level 5 bill would find it odd if the RFV is something simple like toe pain, and it would appear that a level 5 workup was unnecessary. Theoretically, the RFV should warrant a certain amount of workup that then matches up to the final diagnosis. In real life, patients do bring up additional complaints that warrant a bigger workup than what was reported initially, and vice versa, sometimes the RFV seems much more dangerous than the final diagnosis. If the toe pain was actually a necrotic and infected toe related to uncontrolled diabetes, a level 4 or 5 could be warranted, so long as the history, physical, orders,

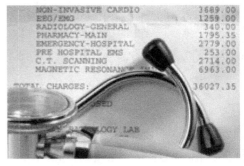

and MDM make that clear. Similarly, if 60 minutes of time is documented for toe pain, the documentation should explain why. Some payers may consider an ER visit "unnecessary" for a particular RFV or final diagnosis and restrict full reimbursement, so again the documentation is essential to prevent possible insurance denials.

Payers also make sure that anything that was billed for is included in the orders and note, essentially meaning that they want to see the physician ordered everything that was done and reviewed it. Forgetting to document the chest Xray order and interpretation in the note might mean that the facility will not get paid for it. Remember the golden rule – if it isn't documented, it didn't happen. So if the physician doesn't document the interpretation of a test, then the physician didn't review it. Hence, the test was not really necessary if the physician did not even bother to look at the results. Results review and interpretation is not only essential for patient care, but also to demonstrate that the test was of value.

At times payers will return discrepancies to the facility to allow for a correction, and this is generally completed through the Health Information Management (HIM) department. The provider will get messages in the EHR inbox identifying chart deficiencies, and it is usually a frustrating process to go back through notes to make corrections and fill in missing information for visits that might have been months ago. Good scribing, however, should eliminate chart deficiencies!

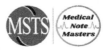

Procedure Documentation and Billing

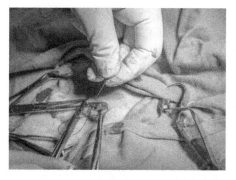

Documenting laceration repairs, fracture reductions, abscess drainage and other procedures are prevalent tasks you will perform as a scribe. Proper documentation for procedures done in the emergency department is essential both for patient safety as well as billing. In addition to the E/M level, procedures are assigned CPT codes for reimbursement. CPT stands for Current Procedural Terminology, a system copyrighted and maintained by the American Medical Association, which assigns numbered codes to all medical procedures, much like ICD-10 assigns codes to diagnoses. Any procedures personally performed by the provider are specially documented as procedures in your note. Anything else, such as procedures performed by a surgeon in the ED, are noted in the Clinical Course, but they are not documented in the provider note as described here.

In most cases, the EHR will have a procedure note template that lists the fields to be completed. In the example laceration note below, several elements are required from a patient care perspective, but also the location and length of the laceration are needed to assign the correct CPT code.

Date, Time Procedure Note, Abscess I&D
Performed by: self *(procedures by residents/students require an attending supervisory note)*
Indication: fluctuant abscess left axilla
Consent: verbal per pt. discussed risks of scarring, continued infection, intrusion into deeper tissues and patient consents to continue
Meds given: 2 cc 1% lidocaine with epinephrine
Procedure: area cleansed with chlorhexidine, then draped. Incision made over area of maximal fluctuance, in parallel with skin fold. Immediate return or malodorous purulent discharge. Pressure applied to encourage drainage, then loculations broken down with a hemostat. 10 cc syringe of saline used to irrigate the cavity. 1/4" packing loosely placed, extruding 2cm, then taped and bandaged with gauze.
Complications: none. Patient tolerated well.

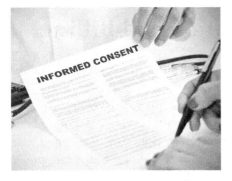

In this case, extensive documentation of consent was not included, since it is a simple procedure on an awake, adult patient. More extensive procedures that involve more potential risk are likely to have a separate consent form, either on paper or in the EHR, that documents more specifically the risks, benefits, and alternatives that were discussed, and that the patient accepts the risks. Some clinics/facilities choose to utilize consent forms more frequently than others, since clear documentation is a good approach to minimize malpractice risk. If your provider reviews risks and benefits with the patient verbally or on a form, the scribe should carefully document the discussion and indicate if a formal paper consent was signed.

EKG billing

Some facilities send all EKGs elsewhere to be formally interpreted, but the provider often interprets the EKG immediately after it is performed, since it may reveal findings that need urgent attention. To bill for EKGs, three findings must be present in the documentation of the EKG interpretation. These will often consist of a combination of the following: rate, rhythm, axis, intervals,

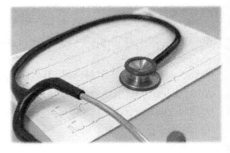

presence or absence of ST-segment changes, and other findings. For example:

EKG: Normal sinus rhythm. Normal axis. No acute ST changes.

Smoking Cessation

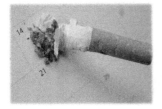

Spending the time to discuss smoking cessation is beneficial to the patient and can be reimbursed if adequately documented. Topics discussed should be specified (think of the 5 A's outlined previously), as well as documentation face-to-face time of >3 minutes or >10 minutes. It also requires documentation that the patient was given instructions and resources for smoking cessation efforts. Entering a diagnosis of nicotine dependence seals the deal.

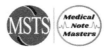

Ultrasound Billing and Documentation

As opposed to ordering a US in the radiology department, physicians may find it necessary to quickly perform a bedside ultrasound for emergent cases or simply for convenience. There may be an EHR template in place already, but generally the elements are similar to those below:

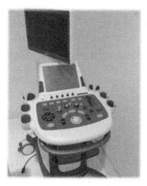

Procedure: Limited Transabdominal Pelvic Bedside US
Indication: +UPT, vaginal bleeding
Performed by: [self]
Procedure: Brand portable US with rounded probe and gel was applied to suprapubic area.
Findings: IUP +FHT
Images are uploaded to the patient chart.

CMS Quality Measures and Reimbursement

For years, healthcare providers were graded on the Physician Quality Reporting System (PQRS). This system set forth well-supported healthcare measures, followed by a process for reporting meeting those measures, and then tied that to reimbursement. In many cases, these measures would be considered standard of care. For example, any female within child-bearing age that presented with a chief complaint of abdominal pain was expected to have a pregnancy test. For patients diagnosed with pneumonia, it is anticipated that oxygen saturation is recorded. Initially, healthcare systems received a bonus for achieving and reporting these measures, but over time, systems that did not correctly report these criteria were penalized. Then in 2017, a new model was adopted to tie reimbursement to quality reporting further: the Quality Payment Program (QPP).

The majority portion of the QPP is called MIPS: Merit-based Incentive Payment System. As the name implies, providers are financially incentivized to meet preset quality measures to be eligible for full reimbursement and avoid penalties. Much like the old PQRS model that it is replacing, QPP provides either positive fee adjustments or penalties (negative fee adjustments), based on reporting the performance of quality measures.

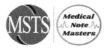

8. Summary

Each practice selects specific measures to track and report on a quarterly or annual basis. Meeting the QPP criteria has a significant effect on reimbursement: +/- 9% in 2020, so healthcare providers are motivated to document, measure and report. All quality measures are reported as a percentage of the time the measure is fulfilled for patients seen with that diagnosis entered in the EHR. If a measure is NOT done for a particular reason, then documentation of that reason should be evident in the documentation so the practice is not penalized for missing the metric.

The full list of primary care options is shown in Figure 7.2. For example, a family practice provider may select these two measures of acute otitis externa care quality:

1. Acute Otitis Externa (AOE): Systemic antimicrobial therapy - avoidance of inappropriate use. Percentage of patients two years of age and older diagnosed with AOE who were not prescribed systemic antimicrobial therapy. Because otitis externa can be fully treated with topical (otic) preparations, it is poor medical practice to treat with a systemic antibiotic, which poses a greater risk of side-effects (e.g., diarrhea) and contributes to the rise of antibiotic-resistant organisms.

2. Acute Otitis Externa (AOE): Topical therapy. Percentage of patients two years of age and older diagnosed with AOE who were prescribed topical antimicrobials.

Health Condition Management Topics within the Quality Measures (continued):

- Sinusitis care including appropriate use of antibiotics and computerized tomography
- HIV viral load suppression
- Pain management for patients in palliative care
- Depression remission
- Adherence to antipsychotic medications for patients diagnosed with schizophrenia
- Asthma control and medication management
- Osteoporosis management for women that have experienced a fracture
- Statin therapy for the prevention and treatment of cardiovascular disease
- Optimal control for ischemic vascular disease
- Appropriate use of antimicrobial therapy for patients with otitis

Opioid Topics within the Quality Measures:

- Opioid therapy follow up evaluation
- Documentation of signed opioid treatment agreement
- Evaluation/interview for risk opioid misuse
- Pharmacotherapy continuity for patients diagnosed with opioid use disorder

Clinician Topics within the Quality Measures that Support Patient Safety and Efficiency:

- Advance care planning
- Document current medications and high-risk medication management
- Communication with the physician or other clinician and closing the specialty referral loop

Figure 7.2: Available MIPS quality measures for primary care (updated 2020)

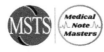

Patient Screening Topic within the Quality Measures:

- Suicide Risk Assessment
- Urinary incontinence assessment with plan of care
- Immunization/vaccination assessment for children and adults
- Screening for breast, colorectal, and cervical cancer
- Eye exam, nephropathy screening test, peripheral neuropathy evaluation, and neurological evaluation for patients with diabetes
- Body Mass Index (BMI) screening and follow up
- Depression screening and follow-up
- Falls screening, risk assessment and plan of care
- Elder maltreatment
- Functional assessment
- Screening for tobacco use with tobacco cessation for adults and adolescents, unhealthy alcohol and brief counseling
- Tuberculosis prevention for patients on a biological immune response modifier for psoriasis

- Hepatitis C virus screening for active injection drug users and patients with cirrhosis
- Human Immunodeficiency Virus (HIV) screening
- Appropriate use of DXA scans for women

Health Condition Management Topics within the Quality Measures:

- Hemoglobin A1C poor control
- Beta-blocker and angiotensin-converting enzyme (ACE) Inhibitor or angiotensin receptor blocker (ARB) or angiotensin receptor-neprilysin inhibitor (ARNI) therapy for left ventricular systolic dysfunction (LVSD)
- Antiplatelet therapy for coronary artery disease (CAD) or anticoagulation for chronic atrial fibrillation
- Children diagnosed with pharyngitis received appropriate streptococcus testing
- Appropriate use of antibiotics for adults with acute bronchitis
- Medication management for depression
- Controlling high blood pressure
- Cardiac rehabilitation referral
- Alcohol and drug dependence treatment

Figure 7.2 continued: Available MIPS quality measures for primary care (updated 2020)

For the emergency department, the process is similar whereby each ED physician or group chooses six quality measures to report.

- Performing a Group A Strep test for child patients with pharyngitis
- Avoid prescribing systemic antimicrobial therapy for patients with acute otitis external (AOE)
- Avoid prescribing antibiotics for adult patients with acute bronchitis
- Timing of thrombolytic therapy for adult patients with acute ischemic stroke
- Avoid unnecessary head computed tomography (CT) scan for minor blunt head trauma for children and adults
- Determine pregnancy location with ultrasound for pregnant patients with abdominal pain
- Follow-up plan for adults screened for high blood pressure
- Adult sinusitis: overuse of antibiotics and CT, appropriate choice of antibiotic
- Utilization of CT for minor blunt head trauma for pediatric and adult patients

Figure 7.3: Available ED MIPS quality measures (Updated 2020)

For the pregnancy location measure example from this list, if every single pregnant patient with abdominal pain has an ultrasound (US) documented, then it can be reported as 100% met. If the patient already had an US that confirmed pregnancy location, the quality measure is met without requiring another US, so documentation regarding the previous US explains why an US was NOT done during today's visit, and the quality measure is still met. As another example, in a patient with a minor head injury, your advance knowledge of this quality measure will reinforce the importance of documenting a thorough MDM regarding why a head CT was done or not done, knowing in advance that the issue will be reviewed.

Another 25% of the QPP score replaces what was previously called Meaningful Use (MU), a system that attempted to promote the use of EHR in a "meaningful" way. Now, these measures are part of the QPP Advancing Care Information (ACI) group. The overall goal of the ACI category is to improve the ability to collect patient data for public health records, limit preventable mistakes, and increase the ease with which patient information can be disseminated to the patient and outside facilities caring for patients. Most notably, it measures an EHR's ability to provide:

1. Security of patient information
2. e-Prescribing of medications
3. Patient access to health information
4. Health information exchange to other clinicians
5. Secure messaging with patients
6. Medication reconciliation
7. Patient-specific educational resources
8. Immunization reporting
9. Other public health reporting

In summary, the QPP/MIPS/ACI has supplanted previous systems (PQRS and MU) to define further how quality reporting and reimbursement are linked. Based on the results from this new system, providers are either given a positive or negative fee adjustment for all Medicare payments which is as high as +/- 9%.

The Joint Commission (TJC) Core Measures

The Joint Commission (TJC), formerly called the Joint Commission on Accreditation of Healthcare Organizations (JCAHO, pronounced "jay-coh"), is a governmental organization that accredits many hospitals and other healthcare organizations.

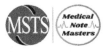

TJC performs physical inspections of both hospitals and EDs every few years. It is imperative to pass this inspection for recredentialing, so an upcoming inspection can lead to a great deal of staff stress. TJC inspections involve direct observation and questioning of ED and hospital physicians and personnel. You should defer to your physician or management if you are present during one of these inspections.

TJC also has their own quality measures, which overlap somewhat with MIPS. Some of these measures involve time from arrival to admit, time from arrival to transfer, and similar times that are not based upon the medical documentation. Like CMS, TJC changes ED Core Measures from time to time so you may need to keep up-to-date. Also, many inpatient quality measures overlap with ED care, such as:

- OP-23 Head CT or MRI Scan Results for Acute Ischemic Stroke or Hemorrhagic Stroke Patients Who Received Head CT or MRI Scan Interpretation Within 45 minutes of ED Arrival
- CSTK-01 National Institutes of Health Stroke Scale (NIHSS Score Performed for Ischemic Stroke Patients)

Billing and Reimbursement Summary

Scribes trained on billing and coding can significantly contribute to the clinic's financial well-being by making sure documentation meets guidelines for billing and quality. Taking the extra time to build useful note templates eliminates the need to memorize these criteria and will save time and dollars in the long-run. Naturally, the note is limited by what the physician actually asks and does with the patient in the clinic, but a good scribe captures and documents those actions in a thorough and organized way, such that the billing and quality measures are crystal clear.

It is not the job of the medical scribe to determine the level of charges, but it is helpful to know why documentation templates are built the way they are, and why certain items are asked and documented. Scribes should have the E/M levels foremost in mind when building EHR note templates at a new job, and consider keeping cheat sheet notecards in your pocket for quick reference. Keep in mind the number of elements listed is the *minimum* requirement, not the goal.

You probably never suspected that your documentation was subject to so much scrutiny! This chapter should give you some idea of what goes on behind the scenes

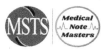

when documentation is being analyzed for various elements. It may also give you some insight into why comprehensive documentation can make such a difference, not only for the direct patient care that day, but also the financial stability of the clinic and broader quality assessments.

$ **Build EHR templates to include E/M level considerations**
$ **The MDM is clinically and financially the most important piece of the note**
$ **Track time, insert placeholder as needed**
$ **Every test ordered should have an interpretation**
$ **Don't make payers question if the workup was necessary**
$ **Procedures are billed separately and require specific separate documentation**
$ **Be aware of quality measures at your institution**

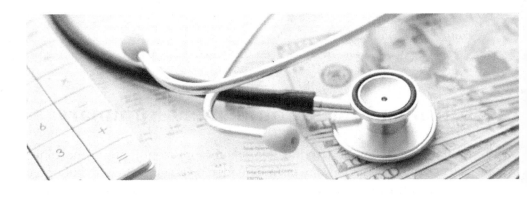

End of Chapter Quiz

1. True or False: an E/M level of 5 has a moderate level of complexity.
    a. True
    b. False
2. How many systems must be listed in the ROS for an ER E/M level 5?
    a. 1
    b. 2
    c. 8
    d. 10
3. Which of the following cannot be counted within critical care time?
    a. Trauma
    b. Respiratory failure
    c. Intubation procedure
    d. Acute MI
4. Documenting an EKG interpretation as "normal" is billable.
    a. True
    b. False
5. Since the 2021 outpatient clinic E/M guidelines no longer count elements in the history, it is OK to just write a sentence or two and skip the rest.
    a. True
    b. False
6. Quality measures promote quality care without financial consequence.
    a. True
    b. False
7. Providers can bill the E/M level OR a procedure from a single encounter, but not both.
    a. True
    b. False
8. Patients understand that procedures have risks, so consent is not needed.
    a. True
    b. False

Answers: 1. B 2. B 3. B 4. B 5. B 6. B 7. B 8. B

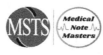

8. The Medical Note Big Picture

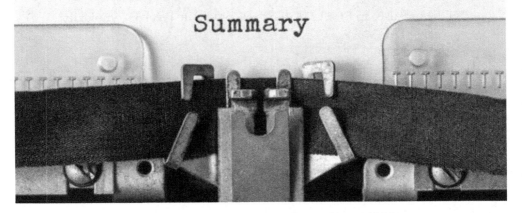

Summary

Throughout this handbook, we have covered a lot of material regarding medical language, the mechanics of the medical note, how to collect and assemble information, and how that information is later analyzed. A thorough note accurately captures today's visit – the story, exam, workup, assessment and plan – in a standardized fashion that is clear for future readers who have various perspectives. In this training, we intend to teach not only the mechanics of compiling the note, but also the purposes of the documentation. With this knowledge, you will understand the broader importance of medical documentation, which will serve you throughout your healthcare career.

The "Note" vs. the "Chart"

A patient's note and chart may sound similar, but they are not the same. The medical note is just one part of the patient's overall "chart." The larger chart contains entries from a wide variety of patient care providers and administrators alike, whereas the note is only the provider's documentation. A provider's note cannot possibly include all of the information from the chart, and likewise, the provider cannot possibly review all of the information contained in the chart. Hence, the note should pull in relevant information from the larger chart (such as vital signs) and specify what the provider has reviewed (such as the social history reported to the nurse). Like old paper charts, the EHR collects large amounts of data over time, and like

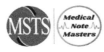

paper charts, the amount of data can be so voluminous that finding information is difficult.

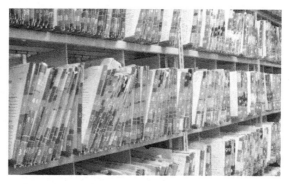

There are far too many EHRs to provide training on all of them, but your future employer's IT department will likely have training material for you to complete before logging in on your first day. Learning to navigate the EHR is essential to performing the majority of healthcare roles nowadays, but EHR companies generally do not provide free training courses nor an online practice environment. If you want to do some prep work before your first day, check out online YouTube videos or similar postings to get an idea of how your new EHR will function.

In addition to navigating the EHR, you need to be a quick typist and mouse clicker to record the clinical findings contemporaneously with the visit. If you are not currently the fastest typist, try out free online typing classes that will, again, benefit you considerably long-term. As soon as you have EHR access, taking the time to

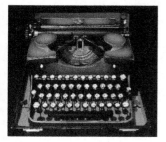

learn some built-in shortcuts will save you time and help you avoid common errors and omissions. In most cases, you can type out a "macro" phrase in advance and then type a short abbreviation in the note to pull in the phrase. For example, you might type up the scribe attestation as follows, then set the abbreviation as ".SCRIBE" such that each time you type. ".SCRIBE" into the provider note, the full attestation macro is entered.

I, Jane Doe, am serving as a scribe to document services personally performed by Michael Smith, MD, based upon my observations and the provider's statements to me. The provider is responsible for reviewing all documentation prior to signing.

I, Michael Smith, MD, hereby attest that this medical record entry accurately reflects signatures/notations that I made in my capacity of physician when I treated/diagnosed the above-listed patient. I do hereby attest that this information is correct, accurate, and complete to the best of my knowledge.

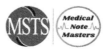

Similarly, you can set up a macro for a routine physical exam or a whole visit note with the appropriate number of elements for billing already set up. When templates and macros are utilized heavily, notes can, unfortunately, begin to look a lot alike – a phenomenon called note cloning. This arises from a lack of attention to the individual details of each patient visit, which a good scribe avoids doing. A similar phenomenon called "note bloat" arises when the note is filled with too much raw data pulled in from the chart, making the note just pages of chart data with only a few pieces of thought-out documentation.

Now that you've polished up your typing and EHR skills, it's time to start scribing!

Today's Visit

HPI Take-Home Points

Although the patient may not cohesively provide the history, remember to keep the narrative organized. If needed, make yourself a notecard or other reminder to keep at your side so that you remember the basic outline and OPQRSTA elements.

- The first sentence sets the stage with immediately pertinent history, age of the patient, and chief complaint(s).
- The second sentence goes back to how this story began.
- The next sentence outlines how the story progressed.
- Generally, pertinent positives are in the HPI body.
- End with pertinent negatives and miscellaneous information.
- Include everything the provider asks.
- Don't forget to include history source(s) and limitations.

Physical Exam Take-Home Points

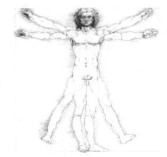

The physical exam goes quickly, so similarly to the HPI, it is wise to make a template of what your provider commonly does – either in the EHR or on a notecard, so you can quickly jot down findings in each system.

Remember that while using macros and EHR templates can save a lot of time, you must make sure to review anything prefilled from

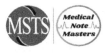

EHR links or entered in a macro. It is relatively easy to enter a normal physical exam template for every patient and to pay attention only to the one system related to the chief complaint, i.e., only altering the musculoskeletal system in an ankle pain patient. This practice, unfortunately, leads to errors of commission in the exam, which should be an objective portion of the note.

If vital signs are pulled in from the chart or documented as reviewed, do not make the mistake of assuming that they are within normal limits. Common typing errors while entering vitals in one area of the chart carries over into the physician's note, and the physician is responsible for those numbers. If, on the other hand, a vital sign is recorded correctly as either low or high, then the physician should address that in the Clinical Course or CDM. For example:

> *Clinical Course: initial HR recorded as 110; however, patient reports running in from the parking lot on a hot summer day. On reassessment, HR is 80.*

While it may seem straightforward, avoid the common mistake of mixing up left and right. Obviously, it's not that you don't know left from right, but it can

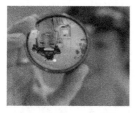

be confusing when the doctor is facing the patient, and the scribe may be facing a different direction. The note should explicitly indicate the location and laterality of each area examined — rather than assuming that the area(s) examined is the same location as the chief complaint.

Assessment and Plan Take-Home Points

The A&P seems as though it would be challenging for anyone other than the provider to document, but most elements are verbalized at one point or another in front of the patient or in related conversations. In particular, pay attention to what the provider explains to the patient and family and convert that into medical terms for the note. Some providers explain more of the MDM than others, so work together with your

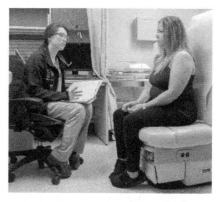

provider regarding the thought process, which is required for documentation but also valuable for your learning process.

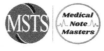

† Don't forget to include the interpretation of data, since interpretation is what turns data into information. EVREYTHING ordered should be interpreted. It is inadequate to write only that the provider saw the CBC results; instead, it is informative to indicate that the CBC results were reviewed, and no significant abnormalities were seen. Indeed, if results are included in the note or marked as reviewed, and they are abnormal, then the note seems quite remiss if an interpretation is not included. For instance:

> A patient's creatinine returns abnormally elevated at 2.5, and labs are marked "reviewed" but without interpretation. Luckily the patient has a lab printout from last year where the creatinine was 2.6, so today's result is stable. Without documentation, it appears the physician neglected the abnormal lab. Further, if a diagnosis of N18.9 Chronic Renal Insufficiency is entered, substantiation regarding chronicity would be lacking.

† In addition to test results, any other investigation the provider did should be included in the Clinical Course or CDM, even if they seem like commonplace tasks. Not only do these pieces of information contribute to the overall assessment, but they count as points toward CDM/MDM complexity.

† Assessments/diagnoses should be as specific as possible. The provider may express the diagnosis directly to the patient, but if not, you may need to ask questions to make sure you select the most appropriate diagnoses from the list of possibilities presented by the ICD-10 list in the EHR. Also, remember the difference between symptoms and diagnoses, since diagnoses are preferred whenever possible. At times no single discrete etiology is identified, and a symptom may be entered as the diagnosis until further workup can be done to pin it further down.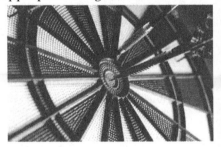

† Include any chronic or background diagnoses that may have been discussed or considered. If a patient presents with chest pain, and uncontrolled hypertension was part of the medical rationale for admission, then it is reasonable to include that in the diagnosis list even though it was not diagnosed today. Most EHRs enable the user to further describe diagnoses as active, inactive, resolved, acute, chronic, etc. and frequently used diagnoses can be saved as "favorites."

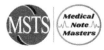

Code	Diagnosis
250.00	Type 2 diabetes mellitus
E11.9	Type 2 diabetes mellitus
O24.111	Type 2 diabetes mellitus affecting pregnancy in first trimester, antepartum
O24.112	Type 2 diabetes mellitus affecting pregnancy in second trimester, antepartum
O24.113	Type 2 diabetes mellitus affecting pregnancy in third trimester, antepartum
O24.119	Type 2 diabetes mellitus affecting pregnancy, antepartum
648.03	Type 2 diabetes mellitus complicating pregnancy, antepartum
250.00	Type 2 diabetes mellitus in patient age 6-12 years with HbA1C goal below 8

Selected Assessment(s)

Code	Diagnosis
E11.9	Type 2 diabetes mellitus

Figure 8.1: Choosing an assessment in an EHR

Narrowing the Differential

As the note progresses, the information collected gradually makes the list of likely etiologies smaller and smaller. Based on the chief complaint alone, thousands of possible etiologies could be at play. After the first sentence and HPI, some possibilities will be considered much less likely. For instance, the chief complaint of "chest pain" will be much less likely to be a heart attack if the patient is 19 years old and has had symptoms constantly for six months. As the note continues and more information is learned, the possible diagnoses will continue to be narrowed down as well. Once you get to the end, those thousands of original possible etiologies will likely be pared down to just a few remaining reasonable possibilities. A well-written note will help in the understanding of this differential narrowing for not only the provider who is seeing the patient today, but for anyone who may need to review the note in the future.

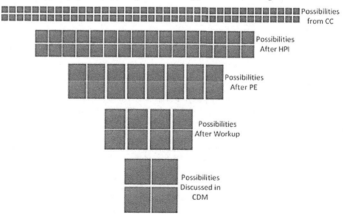

Figure 8.2: Narrowing the differential

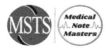

222

Future Readers

We've now achieved our primary goal of investigating the patient's reason for visit, performed a history and physical, diagnosed the problem, and explained the plan. The scribe has documented all that has transpired; the provider reviewed the note and has placed an electronic signature, so our charts are done and mentally set aside as completed. But really, what we've done is sent the note off to a second life, being reviewed by revenue and quality specialists, insurance companies, auditors, ancillary patient care staff, other physicians, and sometimes the patient. With this being the case, clear and accurate documentation is incredibly necessary and should not be taken lightly.

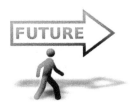

Patient Access

Before the EHR era, patients were able to request a copy of their records, but it was a tedious undertaking that often resulted in a colossal paper printout. With the advent of EHRs and the Meaningful Use program, it became a priority to allow patients easier electronic access to information. The vast majority of EHRs now have a patient access "portal" whereby a patient can sign up for online access and view portions of the chart in a patient-friendly format. Besides portal access, patients can still receive a copy of their chart after signing a release form, but they can now receive full records electronically (with encryption). An example portal is pictured below, where the patient can click on various icons to see test results, active medications, etc. A diagnosis or problem list is pulled in based on the ICD-10 codes selected during documentation.

Figure 8.3: Online patient portal snapshot

| MyChart | | Health | Visits | Messaging | Billing | Resources | Profile |

Health Summary

Use the links to jump directly to a section of your Health Summary.

Current Health Issues   Medications   Allergies   Immunizations   **Preventive Care**

Preventive medicine plays an important part in your health and overall well-being. The following procedures are recommended for people of your age, sex, and medical history.

Overdue

Cholesterol check
Overdue
(i) Learn more

Td/tdap Adults
Overdue
(i) Learn more

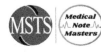

In April 2021, the 21st Century CURES Act was passed which further strengthened patient access to medical records. The CURES Act mandates removal of some systematic barriers to patient access, which results in patients having full access to most medical note types immediately after they are signed. While record transparency has benefits, many

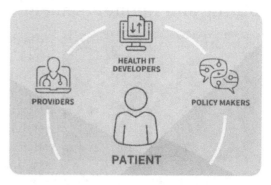

providers are concerned they will need to filter what is documented to avoid causing undue patient anxiety or offense, and that a layperson patient will have difficulty comprehending what is written. Indeed, most students learning medical documentation can relate to that difficulty!

- Some possibly offensive terminology is relatively easy to avoid, such as "SOB" which has another meaning, but generally medical notes are filled with terminology and jargon very difficult for most patients to interpret.
- Providers may discuss various diagnostic possibilities and considerations in the MDM that could be frightening to patients, such as cancer risk.
- The ICD-10 diagnosis code system often uses confusing terms and phrases that do not translate well into plain English.
- Even more confusing are lab and imaging results, which often contain pages of data and numbers that require medical training to interpret.

In either paper or electronic form, anticipate that the patient or family can read, word-for-word, what is written in a signed note. Take care with certain terms, which may not be meant to offend but may not come across well to a non-healthcare provider. One example is something as simple as a "chief complaint" – patients may interpret this as the physician labeling them as "complaining." To stay on the safe side, simply try to avoid possibly offensive terms and be conscientious of your language from a patient's perspective. It is possible over time that some providers or medical documentation practices as a whole will change to be more patient-friendly. Medical documentation already wears a number of hats, and with the CURES Act the patient as a future audience is likely to become a higher priority hat.

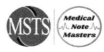

Billing and Reimbursement

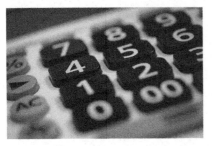

After learning how coding and billing generally work in Chapter 7, you now know the importance of setting up note templates and being thorough in documenting everything that transpires during a visit. CMS does generally set the bar for E/M levels, but there are plenty of other payers that may set more stringent standards, and they all can change over time. The new 2021 outpatient visit guidelines focus on MDM and risk assessment more than "counting beans," but generally, including more discrete, countable elements in the HPI, past histories, PE, and MDM is a plus. Take cues from your provider when possible, since in-house billing personnel will provide providers with billing updates and guidelines intermittently, as well as deficiencies.

Remember that the individual analyzing the note is not a physician and may not even be human! Background processes in the EHR, together with computer-assisted-coding programs, can "count the beans" and determine a preliminary billing level, so omitting elements as "obvious" to a healthcare provider or deviating from standardized note format will be a disadvantage.

The total time spent during the patient encounter (exclusive of separately billed procedures and services) may or not be used by a particular clinical provider. However, the new guidelines make billing by time simpler, so tracking time is likely to be a useful scribe function. In the ER, scribes should prepare to track time for cases that could represent critical care time. Total time is standard practice for telemedicine visits.

Quality Measures

Most quality measures are closely tied to reimbursement and go hand-in-hand with billing concepts. CMS quality metrics are set in conjunction with medical society recommendations and change over time in both content and nomenclature. Healthcare entities that participate in Medicaid and Medicare are financially incentivized to report the CMS guidelines to avoid penalties and to be eligible for full reimbursement percentages.

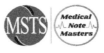

In addition to CMS, other regulatory bodies track quality measures. These also change from time-to-time and depend upon which entity accredits your clinic/institution. Other quality measures may not be tied to reimbursement or regulation at all, such as internal patient care-driven programs that promote appropriate antibiotic use or improving surgical complications.

Knowing which quality metrics are being measured at your particular location is valuable since you can be on the lookout for specific diagnoses or issues that will be included in the measurement. Further, you can use phrases in your documentation that specifically address the quality metric at hand, so that future readers have clarity that the parameter was addressed explicitly rather than needing to read between the lines.

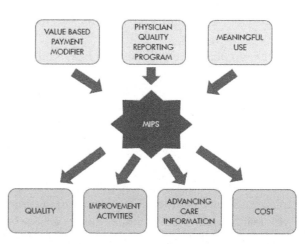

Starting a new position with a provider or clinic has a learning curve, but demonstrating understanding and including quality measures in your template setup will identify you as an advanced documenter.

Medicolegal Aspect

Between 30-55% of physicians will be involved in a lawsuit at some point in their careers, and over time, the fear of malpractice has had numerous effects on medical practice. When it comes to malpractice and documentation, all of our golden rules apply here with one more: avoid regrets! No one wants to look back at a note and wish that something had been written differently. Notes should be written with the presumption that a patient may read it, and the same goes for a lawyer.

Below are two notes for the same patient (subjective sections omitted for brevity). Comparing these two, the events of the visit and E/M levels are similar, yet the notes differ substantially in tone and detail, and thus medicolegal protection.

PE: VS reviewed
GEN: awake alert NAD appears well
HEENT: NC AT
Chest: clear
CV: normal
Extrem: normal
Neuro: alert, ambulatory, cognition clear, facial movements symmetric

A/P: 28 y/o healthy F with tension HA. Neuro intact. POC UPT neg, given Toradol 60mg IM in clinic w/improvement.
Dx: Tension HA
Plan: d/c home. Symptomatic cares.

PE: b/p 120/80 HR 67 RR 14 T99.1 O2 sat 100% RA
Gen: awake, alert, appears well, conversational
HEENT: PERRL without expressed photophobia, EOMI without expressed diplopia. Sinuses nontender. Oropharynx unremarkable, MMM. TMJs nontender. TMs clear. Posterior scalp tender along occipital ridge bilaterally.
Neck: full ROM, tender paraspinal muscles bilaterally, no midline tenderness, no LAD
Respiratory: CTA bilaterally, no increased work of breathing
Cardiovascular: RRR no m/g/r, rate 74
Neuro: CN 2-12 intact, FTN wnl, Romberg neg, no drift. Cognition clear. Ambulatory.

Clinical Course: VSS. POC UPT neg. Administered 60 mg Toradol IM, on reassessment 30" later pt reports feeling better, no adverse reaction.

A/P: 28 y/o F presents with HA x 2 days. History without concerning neuro symptoms or risk factors for SAH. VSS AF. Physical exam findings are benign. Do not suspect intracranial pathology at this point, head CT not indicated by current guidelines, risk of radiation not warranted. D/w pt concerning HA symptoms for which to seek urgent evaluation, including vision changes, cognitive problems, loss of balance or coordination, loss of motor or sensory function, development of n/v, or generally worsening or intractable symptoms.
Dx: G44.209 Tension HA
Plan: d/c home, symptomatic care OTC ibuprofen, consider ergonomics at her desk chair, increase daytime motion and stretching. Initiate HA diary.

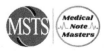

Even with young healthy patients, positive outcomes are not guaranteed and thorough documentation is the best protection against unforeseen circumstances.

Although medical malpractice is usually a provider's biggest concern, the legal system interacts with medicine in other ways as well. Social security disability, car accident litigation, and worker's compensation cases involve special scrutiny of medical documentation. When victims of assault are evaluated, their injuries need careful documentation, including photos when able. Similar above-and-beyond meticulousness is required for child or elder abuse or neglect, since a poorly written note could make a big difference in legal proceedings. Providers may be called to provide a deposition or testimony, and they should be able to look back at the note and recall exactly what transpired.

Summary

Michael Jordan made it look easy, and similarly, a talented physician may seem to diagnose and manage a patient effortlessly. A superficially observant scribe might just document a superficial note, but years of learning, practice, and experience are processed subconsciously during every patient encounter and documentation should reflect that complexity. So, a great documenter follows some golden rules:

If the physician discusses it or does it, document it.

If it isn't documented, it didn't happen.

Avoid regrets.

Knowing in advance how the note will be interpreted in many different perspectives influences the tone of the note and its content. From the physician's perspective today, the note needs to be accurate and medically rational. But then the note takes on multiple personalities as it is viewed by many future readers, each viewing the note with their own needs and own lens in mind. Cognizance of the note's future life can make a good documenter into a great one.

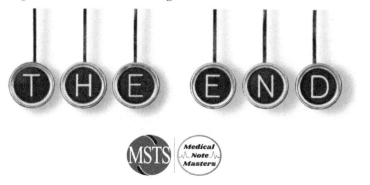

228

Made in the USA
Coppell, TX
14 December 2021

68664622R00134